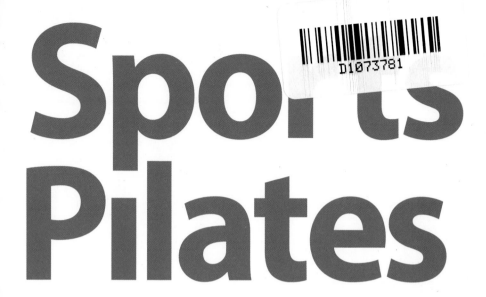

Sports Pilates

How to Prevent and Overcome
Sports Injuries

Paul Massey

Foreword by Peter Blanch, **Australian Institute of Sport**

CICO BOOKS
LONDON NEW YORK

Published in 2011 by CICO Books
an imprint of Ryland Peters & Small Ltd
519 Broadway, 5th Floor,
New York NY10012

Copyright © CICO Books 2004, 2009,
2011

Text copyright © Paul Massey 2004,
2009, 2011

10 9 8 7 6 5 4 3 2 1

A CIP catalogue record for this book
is available from the British Library.

ISBN: 978 1 908170 10 1

Project editor: Charmaine Yabsley and
Marion Paull
Illustrations: Anthony Duke and
Stephen Dew
Design: Jerry Goldie Graphic Design

Printed in China

PUBLISHER'S NOTE:

Always consult a doctor before undertaking any of the advice or exercises suggested in this book. While every attempt has been made to ensure the medical information in this book is entirely safe and correct and up to date at the time of going to press, the Publisher accepts no responsibility for consequences of the advice given therein. If in any doubt as to the nature of your condition, consult a qualified medical practitioner.

THE AUTHOR:

Paul Massey is a leading physiotherapist in private practice and a qualified Pilates Instructor. He has a specific clinical interest in sports injuries, their management and prevention. Massey works closely with governing bodies of track and field, swimming, and field hockey, both at home and internationally, has worked as the Chief Physiotherapist to the Great Britain Swimming Team and has attended numerous Olympic Games, World Championships, and Commonwealth Games in this role. He is also the physiotherapist to the British Athletics English Field Hockey team, British Triathlon team, and Consultant Physiotherapist to the Body Control Pilates Association. He swam the English Channel in 2010. He lectures worldwide on sports injuries and Pilates, and has written a number of books on the subject. He is currently based in Ashford, Kent (UK): visit www.thepartnershipcentre.co.uk for more details.

Contents

Acknowledgments

After years of experience in the sporting area, and in a sports clinic I have seen first-hand the healing benefits of Pilates. After much encouragement, I decided to sit down and share my knowledge: the result is this book. I have been fortunate enough to have had the opportunity to combine physiotherapy and sport, two areas that have provided job satisfaction and ongoing challenges. This book is my way of giving something back. I have many people to thank for making this experience enjoyable and relatively painless:

I wish to take this opportunity to thank my editor, Charmaine Yabsley, whose guidance and support has made this book possible.

I would like to thank CICO books, particularly Mark Collins who believed in me and supported my venture; Cindy Richards who has worked long and hard on this project. We finally got there! May your involvement in Pilates continue even at the end of a long day.

Appreciation also to designer Jerry Goldie for his wonderful designs and Anthony Duke for his inspired illustrations.

There are a number of people who I have worked with over the years who deserve a mention. In particular, Bryan Kennard, who asks the questions to make me think and encourages me to combine the two worlds of physiotherapy and Pilates. Sarah Joyce, who expands and enhances my world of good movement through Pilates, and my patients, from whom I have learned, and continue to learn, so much.

I wish also to mention SD, my family, my sister Anne, and my friends, who continue to support me with encouragement and love. My work colleagues at The Partnership in Ashford, Kent for sharing their clinical experience in this project.

And thank you to Body Control Pilates, which taught me the foundations of Pilates and continues to expand and challenge in my mind its application in the clinical and sporting environment.

Foreword

Over the last several years in the domain of Sports Medicine we have come to realize the importance of efficiency of movement. Not only are our top-level athletes fitter and stronger than the average mortal, the best athletes also use their physiological resources more economically. Whether we consider the long, apparently slow, gliding stroke of the Olympic swimmer or the elegant backhand executed by a top-level tennis player, one thing stands out: these athletes make their performance appear effortless. While this book has been set up for specific sports, the principles and exercises outlined can be applied to all sports. The Pilates philosophy is based around the ease and efficiency of movement. The founder, Joseph Pilates, said his goal of physical fitness was the attainment and maintenance of a well-developed body with attachment to the mind to allow us to perform our many tasks naturally, with zest and pleasure. Pilates has been widely adopted by the professional dance community; the aim of the dancers is to develop the lengthened and strong musculature combined with the body awareness that lead to graceful and elegant movement.

Paul Massey has a unique insight into the application of Pilates philosophy because of his wide experience. He is a physiotherapist with extensive Pilates training as well as a long history of treating elite athletes and dancers. He has taken this insight to help break down the common injuries, the important movement elements, and the best rehabilitation strategies for a variety of sports. The application of the principles outlined in this book will help any athlete in his rehabilitation, but, more importantly, their prevention of further injury. This book will be of interest to the professional and amateur sportsperson. Athletes, coaches, and physical educators will find the straightforward explanations of the type and basic management principles of the common injuries suffered in the listed sports informative. Sports medicine personnel who are deeply involved with the rehabilitation of athletes will welcome the practical exercise suggestions to aid them in the management of their clients. This publication is an excellent handbook to help develop the bridges between movement philosophy, sport biomechanics, and injury.

Peter Blanch, Australian Institute of Sport

Introduction

Pilates is more than just another tool for medical practitioners to use when treating injuries. It is a set of principles designed to help improve the quality of movement. It was established more than fifty years ago by Joseph Pilates (1880-1967) and has been utilized to great success ever since. The success lies in the application of the principles of Pilates to movement. This movement can be used by the majority of the population alongside their normal training program. It will enhance their training and improve their reflexes, strength, and stamina. The focus of this book is to show injured sportspeople an alternative way to rehabilitate damaged muscles, ligaments, and/or joints.

This book illustrates common sports injuries that occur in commonly played sports. Within each sporting chapter I cover the common injuries that can occur as a result of playing that particular sport. A detailed self-assessment and immediate and long-term treatment guidelines are provided. At the end of each chapter you will find the recommended Pilates exercises to help heal and prevent further injury. These exercises are shown in their progressive sequence: core, foundation and performance.

This progression is important to prevent reinjury and allow completion of the rehabilitation process (see page 10). The Pilates method is the main component in this rehabilitation as Pilates strengthens the core areas, lengthens the spine, builds muscle tone, and increases body awareness and flexibility. Furthermore, regular practice of Pilates will enhance your performance in sport and help in the prevention of injuries.

Prevention of injury is better than any cure. Keep this in mind and you will have the physical and mental advantage over your sporting opponent. This book shows you the necessary strategies needed to achieve a good prevention program.

I first became interested in Pilates in my search for a tool to help prevent the occurrence of sports injuries, particularly in competitive swimming. At the time I was working with the national swimming team in Australia, and it was during this time that I discovered the advantages of Pilates. I was impressed by its depth: it was much more than just a series of exercises done in a specific order. I was determined to find out more.

At this time the availability of Pilates teachers and any information was limited. The method had developed by Joseph Pilates in New York and gradually drifted out of the city through an apprenticeship-scheme worldwide. The innovations and presence of qualified apprentices in London saw the development of the training organization, Body Control Pilates, in the United Kingdom. This is where my interest has been developed and fed over the years. This learning process has continued and I have established a unique role as a physiotherapist and Pilates instructor. I now have more than a clinic where I see patients: I have a comprehensive and progressive program that allows the application of quality movement to be applied to the sporting environment, with or without the presence of injury.

I have been using the Pilates method in the sporting environment for a number of years. I used it in two ways: as a rehabilitation tool and as a means of performance enhancement. I hope that through the use of this book you will benefit in your recovery from injury and, more importantly, preventing injuries from occurring in the first instance.

Paul Massey

B.A. (Hons), Msc, M.C.S.P., S.R.P.
Chartered Physiotherapist
Pilates Instructor
Chief Physiotherapist to Great Britain Swimming Team (1989–2000)
Attended numerous Olympic Games, Commonwealth Games, and World Championships as a physiotherapist
Physiotherapist to: British Athletics team, English Field Hockey team
British Triathlon Consultant
Consultant to international governing bodies for swimming, track and field, and field hockey
Physiotherapist to Body Control Pilates Association

All About Injuries

Injuries are an inevitable by-product of playing sport. Many injuries are temporary and heal after a period of rest. As Pilates is a nonintrusive sport, it is ideal for healing and preventing injuries through strengthening and lengthening muscles. The injuries that respond best to Pilates are covered in the following chapters.

What is an injury?

An injury occurs when there is a change in the nature of tissue in the body. This may be caused by a breakdown or disruption of tissue, or by the muscles being overloaded.

Factors to consider during an injury:

• What tissue is involved?

• Mechanism of the injury and factors that caused the injury.

• Rate of onset of the injury.

What tissues are involved?

The easiest way to define the involved tissue is to determine whether the injury is of a soft nature (affecting muscles, tendons, or ligaments) or of a hard nature (affecting bones). The majority of sports injuries are soft.

Immediate treatment

Visit a medical practitioner for an accurate diagnosis of your symptoms.

Follow a specific treatment plan to promote healing.

Follow a comprehensive rehabilitation program to encourage a return to normal strength and flexibility.

NB: It's important to stick to your rehabilitation program; otherwise the injury can return or recur, causing further damage.

Types of injuries

Primary injuries

Primary injuries are usually caused by a collision or muscle tears, or through over use or friction to the muscle or tendon.

Secondary injuries

Secondary injuries occur at a site away from the primary injury. They can occur if the previous injury has been mismanaged or the individual returns to sport too soon.

Rate of onset of injury

An injury may occur at a single event. This tends to apply to acute injuries. If the injury lasts for more than six weeks the injury is defined as chronic.

How injuries heal

There are three stages that occur during the healing process:

1. Acute phase

This phase follows the first 72 hours of an injury and usually involves pain, swelling, redness, heat, and loss of function.

2. Repair phase

The repair phase takes place over a period of three days to six weeks. It is important to maintain a pain-free range of motion during this early stage of rehabilitation (see rehabilitation model page 10).

3. Remodeling phase

The final healing phase takes place over a period of six weeks to several months. As the damaged tissue gradually rebuilds strength and ability, there is less stress on the scar tissue which allows it to heal.

Taking time

The amount of time your body takes to heal from an injury, depends on the severity and location of the injury.

Muscles: six weeks to heal

Tendons/ligaments: twelve weeks

Bones/joints: six to twelve weeks

Managing sporting injuries

The first step in managing your injuries correctly is to ensure you receive an accurate diagnosis of the extent and severity of the injury. This is important to aid recovery and prevent an acute injury from becoming worse. Seek the advice of a chartered physiotherapist or osteopath. Throughout this book, symptoms have been given for the most common injuries

sustained in the various sports, although this is not an exhaustive list.

Treatment

Throughout this book, we recommend the mnemonic **P.R.I.C.E.** as a treatment aid. This stands for **P**rotect, **R**est, **I**ce, **C**ompression, and **E**levation.

Protect: Protect yourself from further injury by stopping sporting activity. If the injury isn't too severe, it may be sufficient to tape the injured area or to wear a splint if bony tissue is involved.

Rest: During the first 48 hours the amount of swelling and bleeding around the injury is at its maximum. It's important to modify your activities and/or take complete rest to reduce any further pain or injury.

Ice: The application of ice cools the damaged tissue by contracting the blood vessels. This prevents further bleeding and swelling and allows the healing process to start.

Compression: Applying compression, even a gentle amount, to the affected area will help to control the development or extent of swelling.

Elevation: By placing the injured area above heart level swelling should drain away. Continue for at least 48 hours.

Rehabilitation

Rehabilitation involves preparing the injured tissue and the rest of the body for a return to sporting activity. You should be able to participate as usual provided that you perform your sport correctly. Incomplete or ineffective rehabilitation will increase the risk of a further injury or recurrence.

Rehabilitation model

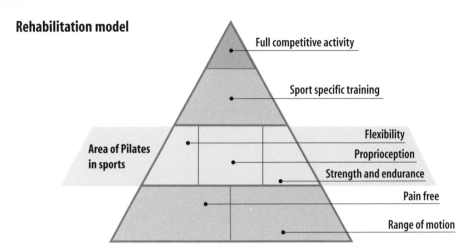

Full competitive activity

Sport specific training

Area of Pilates in sports

Flexibility

Proprioception

Strength and endurance

Pain free

Range of motion

Components of rehabilitation indicating the importance of Pilates

Flexibility

Flexibility is the ability to move a joint of the body through a range of motions. Each joint is designed to allow for a specific amount of motion. The demands of different sports will require a different range of the movement.

Stretching and lengthening

Stretching or lengthening is the method undertaken to achieve length in the muscle (see page 12.)

Benefits of stretching
Improved flexibility

In order for your body to function correctly when undertaking an activity, it is imperative that your muscles are long enough to withstand the required range.

Increased muscle relaxation

During exercise, your muscles will go through a contraction/relaxation process. When undertaking a movement, the muscles on one side of the joint need to release, while the muscles on other side simultaneously contract. This actually allows the muscles to lengthen and relax naturally.

Decreased muscle soreness

Your muscles can become stiff and sore 24 to 48 hours after strenuous activity. They will tend to feel sore and tight and you will most probably experience a restriction in movement, which can affect your training levels.

Improved circulation

Working the muscles will pump the circulation, increasing the flow of blood throughout your body. This helps to improve your performance during exercise, as your mind becomes sharper, reflexes quicker, and muscles stronger.

When to stop

If you feel any sharp pain, numbness, tingling, or burning while lengthening the muscles then stop immediately. There should be some minor discomfort, but this should not last after the exercise has finished. If the pain does continue, you may be working your muscles too hard. You could be exercising too soon after injury, which could cause further damage.

Note: If you are unsure, seek medical advice before continuing.

When to stretch muscles

The best time to undertake lengthening exercise is before and after sport.

How often to stretch

You will need to undertake a specific stretching exercise for the particular muscle you wish to lengthen. This needs to be done regularly to see or feel any benefit. At least two 30-minute sessions per week will help.

Technique

Before beginning any stretching or lengthening, it is important to establish your core areas. That is, pelvis for the lower limb muscles, shoulder blades for the upper limb muscles, trunk for the abdominals (see principles of centering on page 160.)

Lengthening method

1. Move the muscle to its lengthened position. Hold the position for a short period. Feel the muscles extend and become longer. Return to the starting position. Repeat at least 15 times in a slow and controlled way.

Exercises to stretch your muscles

MUSCLE	Exercise
LOWER BACK	double leg stretch, pelvic stability, scissors
SPINE	curl up, roll downs, side rolls, rolling like a ball, open leg rocker
HAMSTRINGS	double leg stretch, hamstring lengthening, scissors, leg circles, open leg rocker
PSOAS	spinal curls, scissors, swimming
QUADRATUS LUMBORUM	hip opening, spinal curls, side reach
HIP ABDUCTORS	big squeeze, roll downs
HIP ADDUCTORS	leg circles, hip opening, open leg rocker
QUADRICEPS	single knee kicks, swimming
GLUTEALS	mid back stretch, open leg rocker
PIRIFORMIS	hip opening
HIP ROTATORS	leg circles, single knee kicks
TIBIALIS ANTERIOR	heel drop, tennis ball raises
GASTROCNEMIUS	roll downs
SOLEUS	roll downs, wall slides
RECTUS ABDOMINIS	dart
OBLIQUES	superman, spinal curls
LATISSIMUS DORSI	double leg stretch
PECTORALIS MAJOR	double leg stretch, arm opening
PECTORALIS MINOR	arm opening
TRAPEZIUS	mid-back stretch, shoulder external rotation, shoulder internal rotation
ANTERIOR DELTOID	double leg stretch, wall slides, threading the needle
POSTERIOR DELTOID	threading the needle
BICEPS	dart
TRICEPS	arm circles
NECK FLEXORS	diamond press, dart
NECK ROTATORS	neck rolls, roll downs
ACHILLES TENDON	tennis ball raises, heel drop
WRIST FLEXORS	wrist openings
WRIST EXTENSORS	wrist openings

2. Identify the muscle that needs to be lengthened. Identify the Pilates exercise that will work the muscle into a lengthened position. Follow the instructions for that exercise.

N.B. It is necessary to undertake preparation exercise before you attempt any performance exercises. Incorrect preparation may result in a torn or pulled muscle.

If the tissue is actively inflamed and the area is hot, red, or swollen, do not attempt any exercise. Similarly, if there is an open cut to the skin, lengthening may reopen the wound and delay healing. An injured muscle or joint may need an assessment by a medical practitioner before beginning any lengthening exercises, in order to prevent further damage.

Strengthening

Program for strength training

Complete the core exercises (page 169) before graduating to the foundation exercises (page 179). It's important to complete both of these before moving on to the performance exercises. Concentrate on the exercises that strengthen the specific muscle you are focusing on for training.

Complete a comfortable number of reps. The reps should be slow and controlled without any rest between them.

Maintain the quality of the movement. Stop if you lose your technique.

When you can complete approximately twenty reps of an exercise, aim to perform a second set of that exercise.

Start with two specific training sessions for your selected area per week and build

What you should lengthen or strengthen according to your sport

TENNIS, BASEBALL

Shoulders, arms, back, hamstrings, quadriceps, calves.

SWIMMING

Shoulders, arms, back, neck, legs.

RUNNING

Back, hips, groin, quadriceps, hamstrings, calves.

FOOTBALL, SOCCER

Back, hips, groin, quadriceps, hamstrings, calves.

CYCLING

Back, quadriceps, hamstrings, calves.

WEIGHT TRAINING IN THE GYM

Back, shoulders, hips, forearms, thighs.

SKIING AND SNOWBOARDING

Quadriceps, hamstrings, hips, calves, back.

SAILING AND WINDSURFING

Arms, back, quadriceps, shoulders.

HORSE RIDING

Back, hips, quadriceps, hamstrings.

GOLF

Trunk, back, hips, quadriceps, hamstrings, calves, shoulders.

up to three per week. Have a day off between each session. Work on another area that is used in your sport but does not relate to your injury.

After about 12 weeks you should be comfortable enough to undertake three sessions per week. Do three sets of approximately twenty reps of each exercise.

Note: As you build up muscle strength you will find that you experience muscle soreness. As long as this soreness is not too painful, continue with your training.

Proprioception

A good presence of proprioception ties in closely with the principles of Pilates: smooth coordinated movements that flow and can be repeated over and over in a correct sequence. Proprioception helps to build concentration and focus, enabling the mind to achieve a sense of lengthening and strengthening of the muscles.

Proprioception training is highly common during the rehabilitation of injured athletes, but it can just as easily be used to prevent injuries.

If the proprioception process is overlooked in the rehabilitation of a sporting injury, or is not used as part of a conditioning program, there is a possibility that the problem may recur. Certainly, performance will be affected. Proprioception training attempts to maximize protection from injury and provide optimal functional restoration.

Factors to remember

Proprioception exercises should begin as soon as possible after injury, but should never create more discomfort.

Exercises should not stress the healing tissue, but enhance the general coordination of the muscles.

Stages of exercise

1. Ability to achieve random movement of the joint without pain.

2. If the joint is able to bear weight, achieve the range with weight exercises.

3. Gradually build up the difficulty of the exercise, reducing the base of support. For instance, close your eyes and reduce the stability of your base by using a wobble board.

Progression: Make the exercises more complicated. Integrate specific drills into your sports to increase your agility and balance.

Four elements of proprioception

1. Joint positional awareness

Involves a functional range of motion in a closed chain position.

Aims

To achieve a sense of balance.

To improve reflex action.

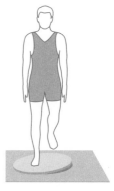

A wobble board is used to challenge balance.

2. Dynamic stabilization

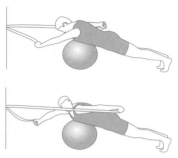

Aims

To complete the dynamic joint stability exercises.

To encourage agonist/antagonist coactivation.

To enhance the force couples arrangement of the muscles around the joints.

3. Reactive neuromuscular control

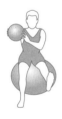 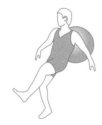

Aims

To focus on the reflex from the joint/muscle receptors to the muscle.

4. Functional motor control

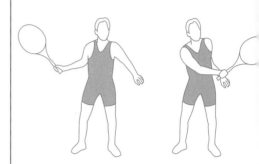

Aims

To return the athlete to pre-injury level of physical strength and flexibility.

To reduce the risk of reinjury.

Checklist before returning to sports

✓ Achieved adequate cardiovascular fitness.

✓ Regained skills specific to your sport.

✓ Corrected any biomechanical problem present that may have contributed to the initial problem.

✓ Established confidence in your ability to return to sports.

✓ Been educated in injury prevention.

Prevention of injuries

Pilates can help reduce the chance of injury through its focus on lengthening, strengthening and proprioception (balance).

Prevention guide

1. Warm up and warm down

Your warm up should reflect the type of activity to be undertaken. For general exercises, the foundation Pilates group (see page 179) is ideal for warming up the entire body. Move on to the performance exercises (see page 204) for a more intensive warm up. Performance exercises should follow only an initial warm up. You should warm up for about 15 to 30 minutes.

2. Lengthening and stretching

A good lengthening program helps maintain the length in the muscle, reduces the onset of muscle soreness, and enhances recovery.

3. Taping and strapping

Taping and/or strapping is used as a protective mechanism during the healing and rehabilitation of tissue.

4. Fitness levels

Don't try to increase your fitness levels all at once. Increase your activity level by no more than ten percent each week. Being a "weekend warrior" (doing all your activity in two days) puts you at risk owing to the intensity of activity. Aim to do at least thirty minutes of exercise each day.

If you are new to exercise, break the thirty-minute goal into three achievable ten-minute sessions.

5. Use appropriate protection

Protective equipment is designed to shield various areas from injury. Protective equipment, such as mouth-guards and shin pads, can also be worn after an injury to protect the area from direct contact.

6. Footwear

Choosing the right sports shoe is determined by your foot type and your requirements. To determine your foot type see the wear pattern (page 16).

7. Recovery program

Don't overdo it. Training too much will lead to sore, tired, and overused muscles. And if you are training incorrectly the problem will only become exacerbated.

8. Don't train when you're tired

If you feel tired your muscles are tired. Tiredness leads to a lack of reflex action which can lead to injury.

9. Maintain good training technique

The way in which you perform an activity can have far-reaching effects on your body. If your technique or movement quality is poor, problems such as muscle imbalances can arise (see page 134).

10. Stick to the rules of the sport

The rules of every sport are there to protect the players.

How to choose a shoe for your foot type

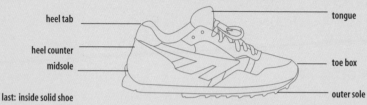

heel tab — tongue

heel counter —
midsole — toe box

last: inside solid shoe — outer sole

Pronators – foot tends to roll inward

Look for: Firm midsole. Board or combination lasting. Straight/slightly curved last. Firm heel counter.

Avoid: Extra soft midsole. Slip lasting. Very curved last. Soft heel counter.

Common injuries: Patellofemoral knee pain. Medial knee pain. Plantar fasciitis. Shin splints. Tibial stress fractures. Lower spine pain.

Supinators – foot tends to roll outward

Look for: Soft midsole. Curved last. Slip lasting. High heel lift.

Avoid: Very firm midsole. Straight last. Board lasting. Thin heel.

Common injuries: Nerve pain behind the toes. First toe pain. Plantar fasciitis. Achilles tendon pain. Iliotibial band syndrome. Heel pain.

Wear patterns on sport shoes indicate problems

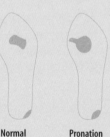
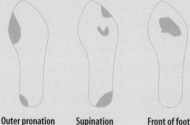

Normal   Pronation   Outer pronation   Supination   Front of foot

11. Treat injuries appropriately

Pain after activity, during the warm up or near the end of your activity session is an early sign of an overuse injury.

Possible training errors:

Sudden increase in training mileage or intensity.

Excessive hill training.

Being unprepared (that is you haven't warmed up correctly) for the activity.

Action to take:

Correct training errors.

Ice the injured part after your training.

Minimize the aggravating part of your training and use cross training (use gym exercise safety) as an alternative if required.

If pain increases with the activity a period of time is required to allow the tissues to heal. Rest or reduce the amount of activity for a few days.

Common gym exercises that create problems

Ballistic toe stretch

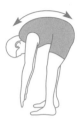

Potential injuries: Can cause injury to the lumbar spine if the disk or muscle is unable to support itself in this position. This can occur if there is more movement in the spine than in the hamstrings when bending during the exercise.

Ballet or hamstring stretch

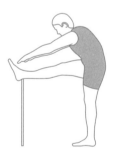

Potential injuries: Can place strain on the ligaments of the lower back or the sciatica. If hamstrings are not flexible or lengthened, they can become overloaded or pulled. If the pelvis moves or rotates during this movement strain can be placed on the sacroiliac joint.

Seated leg stretch

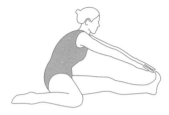

Potential injuries: Strain may be placed on the medial compartment of the knee (ligaments, menisci, medial hamstrings).

Neck circles

Potential injuries: Neck injuries can easily occur during this movement. especially compression of the soft tissues of the cervical spine and strain to the facet joints in the neck.

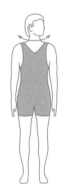

Quadriceps stretch

Potential injuries: Twisting the pelvis as the leg is pulled back can cause a strain on the lower back. The knee of the supporting leg can also become locked.

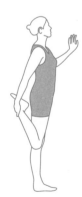

Oblique crunch

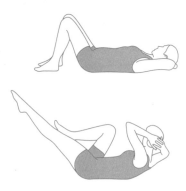

Potential injuries: Excessive rotational strain on the thoracic spine. The neck may become strained if you poke your chin out during the crunch. An incorrect oblique crunch may also cause injury to the ribs or lower back owing to over-rotation.

Straight leg lift

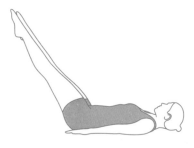

Potential injuries: Poor abdominal control or weakness will lead to strain on lumbar spine. Excessive effort may be made through the ribs and thoracic spine.

Back extensors

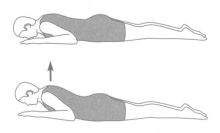

Potential injuries: It is necessary to maintain good trunk control to avoid any movement in the lower back.

Note: If you are unsure whether or not you are performing your exercise correctly, ask a staff member at your gym.

See the chart on page 21 and follow the recommended Pilates program. This program will help to strengthen and lengthen your muscles to help improve performance and prevent injury.

Free weights

Dumb bell chest press

Aim: Works the chest muscles, along with the shoulders and triceps.

Method: Lie on a bench with a weight in each hand, feet up on the bench. Push the dumb bell up so that your arms are directly over your shoulders and your palms are facing forward. Lower the weights down toward your body until your elbows are slightly below your shoulders. Lift the weights and repeat.

Mistakes to avoid: Don't lock your elbows out as you push the weights up. Keep your shoulder blades firmly on the bench; otherwise, you will lose the natural arch in your back.

Pull up

Aim: To work the muscles of the upper back.

Method: Standing underneath a chin-up bar, grab the bar with the palms facing you and hands slightly closer than shoulder-width apart. Bend your arms and lift your chest toward the bar. When your chest reaches the bar, slowly lower back to starting position.

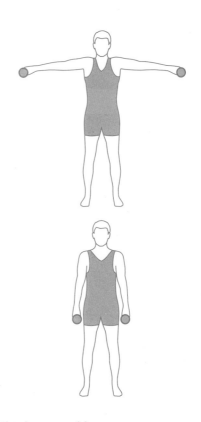

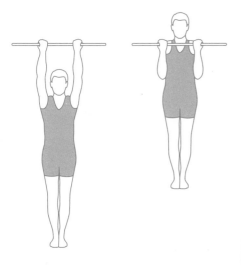

Mistakes to avoid: Don't arch your back or lift your body during the exercise. Keep your shoulders level—don't bring them up toward your ears.

Lateral raise

Aim: Works the deltoid muscles of your shoulder (supraspinatus muscle).

Method: Lift your arms up and out to sides until the weights are just below shoulder height. Lower the weights in a slow, controlled manner.

Mistakes to avoid

Don't lift your shoulders or move your elbows throughout the movement. Use your strength to complete the move, don't arch your back to initiate it. Keep your core steady—don't rock back and forth. Don't raise the weights above shoulder height.

Biceps curl

Aim: Works the biceps, brachioradialis, anterior deltoid, and pectorals.

Method: Sit with your legs crossed, a weight in each hand, with the palms facing inward. Raise one arm up at a time,

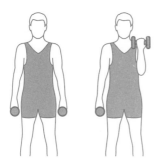

Method: Place your hands on the edge of a flat bench. Rest your feet on the floor in front of you with your knees bent. Bend your arms. Return by straightening your arms to starting position.

Mistakes to avoid:

Don't allow your wrists to bend backward rather than keeping them straight. Keep the hips/back close to the bench throughout the motion. Don't thrust up through the hips.

turning the palm up. Raise your elbow to continue curling the weight.

Mistakes to avoid: Don't lift through the shoulder rather than maintaining a stable base. You may be tempted to lean back in order to complete the move, so focus on your core. Don't lift your elbows out wide, keep them close to your body. Maintain control of the weights during the motion.

Triceps dips

Aim: Works the triceps, pectorals, and anterior deltoid muscles.

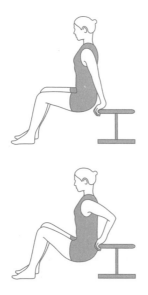

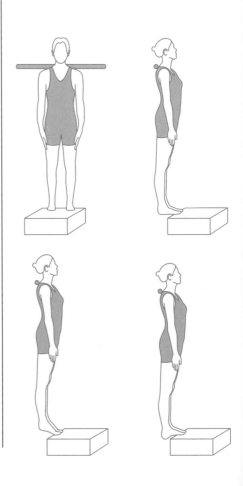

The Pilates alternatives to gym exercises

	Ballistic toe stretch	Ballet or hamstring stretch	Seated leg stretch	Neck circles	Quadriceps stretch	Oblique crunch	Straight leg lift	Back extensors
CORE EXERCISES								
curl up	●							
diamond press				●				
imprinting				●				
pelvic stability							●	
FOUNDATION EXERCISES								
arm circles								
arm opening				●				
dart				●				●
hamstring lengthening	●	●	●					
long sitting stretch	●							
neck rolls				●				
roll downs	●			●				
single knee kicks			●		●			
spinal curls			●					●
wall slides				●				
PERFORMANCE PILATES								
double leg stretch		●	●				●	
oblique curl up						●		
open leg rocker		●	●					●
roll up	●							
rolling like a ball			●					●
scissors	●	●	●					●
single leg stretch		●	●				●	
superman						●		
swimming			●		●			●

Standing calf raises

Aim: Works the gastrocnemius muscle (calf muscle).

Method: Stand with your back straight in front of the machine or bar. Place your shoulders under the weight (machine or bar) and place your toes and the balls of your feet on the toe block. Lower your heels, then rise up as high as you can on your toes while keeping your knees extended. Return to start position.

Resistance exercises with machines

Leg curls

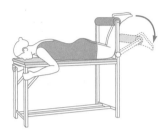

Aim: To involve entire hamstring group.

Method: Lie face down on the machine. Straighten your knees and hook your feet under the set of roller pads. Raise your feet upward until your knees are as bent as possible. Return to starting position.

Mistakes to avoid: Don't lift the hip bones or allow the abdominals to lose control of the pelvis. Don't return to the starting position too quickly. Over-stretching when the bar is above the head may strain the back.

Leg extensions

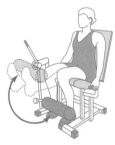

Aim: To localize movement of the quadriceps.

Method: Sitting at the machine, hold the hand grips to steady your body. Bend

your knees and place your ankles under the set of roller pads. Raise your legs until they are almost parallel to the floor. Slowly lower to the starting position.

Mistakes to avoid: Make sure you are sitting correctly before beginning. Don't lock your knees. Arching your back in an effort to help you lift the weight can cause back strain.

Bench press

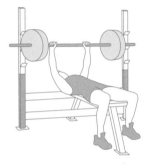

Aim: To focus on the upper body muscles (pectorals and triceps, anterior deltoids, serratus anterior and coracobrachialis).

Method: Lie on your back on a flat bench. Keep your buttocks in contact with the bench and your feet flat on the floor. Take an overhand grip on the bar bell with your hands more than shoulder-width apart. Slowly lower the bar until it reaches your chest. Return to starting position.

Mistakes to avoid: Not breathing correctly: breathe out as you press the bar up, breathe in as you lower it. Don't move around or arch your back in order to lift the weight as this will lead to stress on the lower back. Keep your elbows relaxed and avoid pushing the bar too high. The shoulders should stay in contact with the bench throughout the movement.

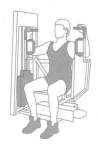

Pec deck

Aim: To stretch the pectoral muscles.

Method: Sit on the machine seat and press your elbows into the pads, relaxing the forearms and wrist action, force the pads together until they touch in front of your chest. Allow the pads to return slowly to the starting position.

Mistakes to avoid: Check your posture regularly to make sure you don't poke your chin forward, as this will place strain on and make you lose the position of your shoulder blades. Make sure you work each side equally.

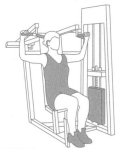

Shoulder press

Aim: To strengthen the muscles around the shoulders.

Method: Push your arms above you in order to extend through the elbows. Lower to starting position.

Mistakes to avoid: Don't arch the lower back as you push upward. Check your posture to make sure you're not poking your chin forward.

Aerobic equipment

Rowing machine

Mistakes

Pulling the bar too low or too high.

Opening your knees on your return to the starting position.

Allowing the bar to bounce off your chest as you pull it toward you.

Leaning back as you pull through the bar.

Shrugging your shoulders and shortening the neck forward.

Bike

Mistakes

Having the seat at the wrong height. See page 49 for advice on the correct position and choosing the right bike.

Allowing the knee to roll while cycling. Keep the knee moving over the direction of the mid-foot as you cycle.

Leaning into the handle bars, which allows the shoulder to elevate and the chin to poke out, creating pressure on the neck.

Treadmill

Mistakes

Allowing the shoulder to tense up and so elevating the shoulders.

Running on your toes. You need to use a heel–toe movement.

Leaning forward to run, which changes your line of gravity. This can lead to strain in the calf muscles.

Not allowing your shoulder to twist opposite to your leg while running— creating a stiff trunk.

Not keeping your eye gaze forward.

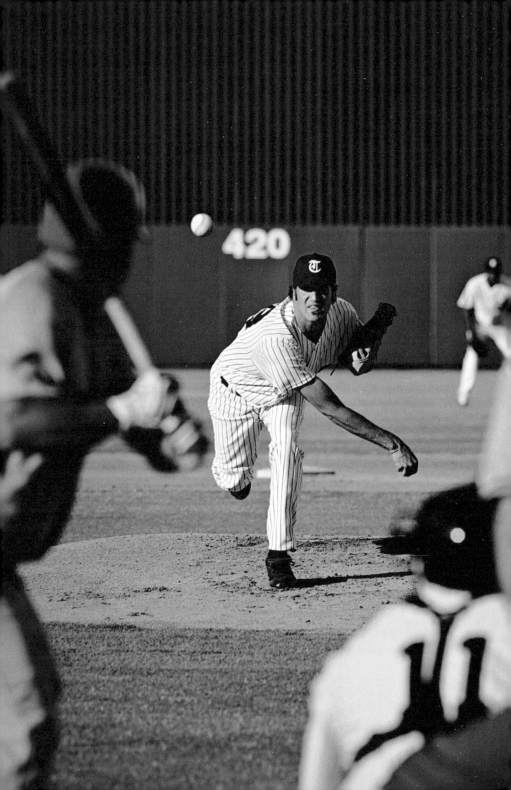

Baseball

Injuries in baseball are usually caused by incorrect technique in the pitching motion, resulting in imbalance in the muscles of the forearm and shoulder. They are generally defined as either cumulative (overuse) or acute (traumatic) injuries. Overuse injuries build up over time due to stress on muscles, joints, and soft tissues. They begin as small, nagging aches or pains, and can grow into debilitating injuries if not treated early or given proper time to heal. Acute injuries are caused by a sudden impact, and can be dramatic.

Common baseball injuries

Rotator cuff pain

This is one of the most common injuries to afflict baseball players, because of the repeated throwing involved in the game—in pitching and fielding.

Causes

Stress and strain on arms and shoulders.

Signs and symptoms

Pain in the front aspect of the shoulder. The pain is usually located in the attachment of the supraspinatus tendon in the shoulder.

Pain in the posterior aspect of the shoulder (infraspinatus attachment). This may indicate a possible partial dislocation (subluxation) of the glenohumeral head (shoulder joint) during activity. Subluxation is excessive shoulder joint movement within the socket of the joint.

Rotator cuff area: sites of pain

Broken collarbone

Shoulder separation

Dislocation

Shoulder impingement

Rotator cuff

Biceps tendonitis

Weakness in the scapular muscles. Weak external rotators in the shoulder and weak abductors.

Treatment

IMMEDIATE

Application of P.R.I.C.E. to the tender area. Limit throwing while pain continues.

Rotator cuff movement tests

Test to indicate balance of rotation around the shoulder.

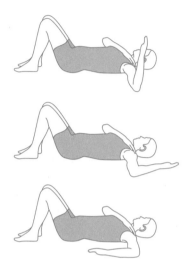

Test for anterior impingement of a rotator cuff muscle.

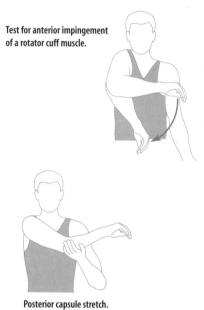

Posterior capsule stretch.

LONG-TERM

Focus on exercises that improve your ability to rotate the internal muscles of the shoulder.

Concentrate on stretching the posterior capsules (see above).

Strengthen the decelerators and scapular stabilizers muscles (rhomboid and serratus anterior).

How to prevent

Check to ensure that you have an internal rotation range greater than 80 degrees while holding your arm at a 90-degree angle to your body.

Spend time concentrating on improving your throwing technique.

Acromioclavicular joint sprain

The acromioclavicular joint (AC) is vulnerable to injury in collision sports and in activities requiring repetitive overhead motions, such as upper-extremity strength training. The key to successful treatment is prompt and accurate recognition of the severity of AC injuries.

Causes

Falling on to your outstretched arm.

Repetitive overarm pitching.

Signs and symptoms

Pain, tenderness or possible deformity around the AC.

Classification of pain

GRADE ONE PAIN

Symptoms: Pain or tenderness.

Treatment: Treat symptoms through P.R.I.C.E. Continue activity.

GRADE TWO PAIN

Symptoms: Pain, tenderness, and slight separation from the prominent end of the clavicle.

Treatment: Use a sling and rest for two to four weeks depending on severity.

GRADE THREE PAIN

Symptoms: Pain, tenderness, and marked separation of the joint from the prominent end of the clavicle.

Treatment: You may need to wear a brace and rest for six to eight weeks. Surgery may be necessary.

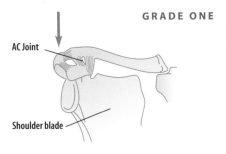

GRADE ONE

AC Joint

Shoulder blade

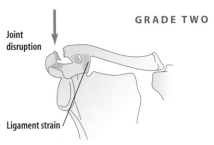

GRADE TWO

Joint disruption

Ligament strain

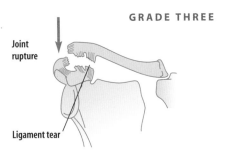

GRADE THREE

Joint rupture

Ligament tear

Diagram of acromioclavicular joint sprain.

Labrum damage

The labrum of the shoulder consists of fibrocartilage tissue around the rim of the shoulder joint. It cushions the bones of the joint and allows good rotation. Baseball players may suffer a tear in the upper labrum, extending from front to back, referred to as a SLAP lesion (Superior Labrum Anterior Posterior).

Causes

Repetitive forceful contraction that compresses the shoulder joint and places great stress on the labrum during the deceleration phase of the throwing motion.

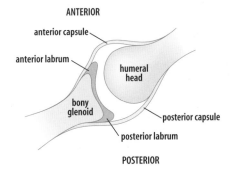

ANTERIOR

anterior capsule

anterior labrum

humeral head

bony glenoid

posterior capsule

posterior labrum

POSTERIOR

Diagram of labrum location

Phases of the overhand pitching used in baseball

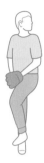 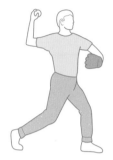 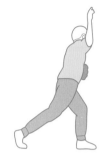

Windup
Balanced and preparation phase in which opposite leg is cocked.

Cocking
Begins as hands part and ends when the throwing arm is in extreme rotation.
Injuries: forearm muscle strain; nerve damage; shoulder instability; labrum tears

Acceleration
Begins when the ball moves forwa with internal rotation of the uppe arm and ends with ball release.
Injuries: muscle strain in forearm; elbow problems; shoulder problem

Signs and symptoms

Localized pain in shoulder, aggravated by overhead motion and extending the arm back. Popping and catching sensation may be present.

Tenderness to front of shoulder joint.

Pain on biceps contraction.

Treatment

INITIAL

Identify cause in pitching action, possibly in deceleration phase.

LONG-TERM

Surgical intervention may be necessary. Seek specialized medical advice.

How to prevent

Learn correct body mechanics of throwing action.

Joint subluxation

In baseball, dislocation, or subluxation, of a joint usually occurs to the shoulder. The top part of the arm bone (humeral head) slips out of its socket (glenoid cavity). When a forward (anterior) dislocation occurs, the labrum (the cartilage that stablizes the shoulder joint) is frequently torn. Shoulder dislocations can also occur backward (posterior) and downward (inferior).

Causes

A dislocation can occur when the arm is forcibly moved into an awkward position during a fall or forced pulling on a joint. If a dislocation, or partial dislocation, occurs when the force seems minor, the injury may be caused by multidirectional instability.

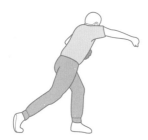

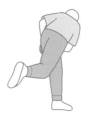

Deceleration

The elbow extends as the shoulder absorbs violent distraction force by contraction of the rotator cuff muscles.

Injuries: biceps strain; olecranon damage; elbow capsular strain; rotator cuff partial tear; biceps tendonitis/rupture; labrum damage; shoulder subluxation

Follow-through

The body moves forward with the arm to relieve tension on the rotator cuff muscles. Strength on the opposite leg controls smooth transition to recovery as the trailing leg contracts the floor.

Injuries: acromioclavicular joint problems; shoulder subluxation

Signs and symptoms

Loss of active range of movement in the shoulder joint in most directions.

Feeling your joint "pop out".

Loss of normal profile or appearance in the shoulder region.

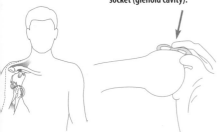

A shoulder dislocation is when the top part of the arm bone (humeral head) slips out of its socket (glenoid cavity).

Site of pain

Joint subluxation

Treatment

IMMEDIATE

Seek medical attention.

Place the arm in a sling for approximately ten days, making sure the elbow does not get stiff and the neck maintains a normal range of motion.

Practice isometric exercising the rotator cuff muscle while in a neutral joint position to help your range of flexibility.

Seek expert advice regarding your rehabilitation in order to prevent a recurrence of the dislocation.

If this is the first time you have dislocated your shoulder, relocation may occur itself.

LONG-TERM

Strengthen the muscle over a period of at least 6 to 12 weeks.

Don't expect full strength to return for six months or more.

Check range of movement in the muscle around the shoulder joint, to check for any muscle imbalances around the joint.

Respect the pain you are experiencing and don't play again until your shoulder heals.

Follow the Pilates program outlined at the end of this chapter.

How to prevent

Maintain good strength and good coordination in the shoulder and rotator cuff area (see page 25).

Biceps tendonitis

Biceps tendonitis is a common injury among athletes who use the majority of their upper body. The symptoms are very similar in appearance to impingement syndrome and the two conditions are often confused. Biceps tendonitis is a result of inflammation of the long head of the bicep at its insertion into the scapular (shoulder blade).

Pain tends to occur when the arm is lifted overhead and the elbow is flexed at greater than 90 degrees to the shoulder.

Causes

Poor technique or repetitive movement can cause this injury. Too much weight-pulling through the arm can exacerbate the problem because the tendon tends to become inflamed in the tendon groove.

Signs and symptoms

Tenderness in the front aspect of the shoulder joint (the biceps groove).

Pain when lifting the arm above the head.

Treatment
IMMEDIATE

Modify the amount of activity to avoid aggravating the pain.

Apply ice to the area.

LONG-TERM

Check the range of movement in the muscles around the shoulder joint. This determines whether there are any muscle imbalances around the joint.

Do not play baseball until you recover.

Follow the Pilates recovery program outlined at the end of this chapter to expedite your recovery.

Check your technique.

Little pitcher's shoulder

This is defined as a Salter 1 type fracture of the proximal humeral growth plate—a fracture through the bone growing plate in upper arm.

Cause

Poor pitching technique.

Signs and symptoms

Shoulder pain is aggravated by throwing.

Pain, nonspecific to shoulder, is worse after activity and hard throwing.

Tenderness in the upper arm (the growth plate area.)

Treatment
INITIAL

Correct diagnosis—X-ray investigation may be required.

LONG-TERM

Six weeks rest from any form of throwing, or even batting, to allow fracture to heal.

How to prevent

Learn correct body mechanics of throwing action to prevent overuse injury.

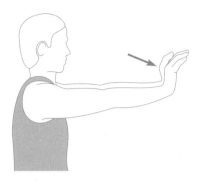

Little leaguer's elbow

This is defined as pain on the inside (medial) aspect of the elbow. A repetitive throwing motion will create valgus stress—tension on the structures on the inside of the joint—and will also cause problems to the medial epicondyle, medial epicondylar apophysis, and the medial collateral ligament. Repeated stress results in overuse injury, when tissue breakdown exceeds tissue repair. In older pitchers, this usually takes the form of damage to the medial collateral ligament.

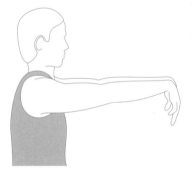

Assessment technique for little leaguer's elbow

Cause

Training errors, such as changes in intensity, duration, or frequency of throwing activities.

Strength and flexibility imbalance in the muscle of the forearm, or in the shoulder musculature.

Damage to the growth plate in the elbow.

Signs and symptoms

Pain on the inside of the elbow.

Pain aggravated by resisted wrist flexion.

Pain aggravated by elbow and wrist extension in supination, i.e. with the palm down.

Treatment
INITIAL
Application of ice

LONG-TERM
Stretching forearm muscles.
Strengthening program.

How to prevent
Learn proper body mechanics of throwing action.

Follow a structured, year-round exercise program.

Strengthen elbow/shoulder concentric and eccentric muscle action.

Pilates exercises to improve performance and prevent further injury

▌ Lengthen
▼ Balance
● Strengthen

	Rotator cuff pain	Acromioclavicular joint sprain	Labrum damage	Joint subluxation	Biceps tendonitis	Little pitcher's shoulder	Little leaguer's elbow
CORE EXERCISES							
curl up				●	●	●	●
diamond press	●	●	●	●	●	●	●
floating arms	●		●	●	●	●	●
four point challenge	▼	▼	▼	▼	▼	▼	▼
static standing balance	▼		▼				
FOUNDATION EXERCISES							
arm circles	●		●	●	●	●	●
arm opening	●	▌	●	▌	▌	▌	
long sitting stretch				●	●	●	●
mid-back stretch	●		●	●	●		
roll downs				●			●
shoulder rotation control		●				▌	●
side reach				●	●	●	●
spinal curls			●				
star				●	●	●	

	Rotator cuff pain	Acromioclavicular joint sprain	Labrum damage	Joint subluxation	Biceps tendonitis	Little pitcher's shoulder	Little leaguer's elbow
PERFORMANCE PILATES							
double leg stretch				■●	■	■●	■●
hundred	●	●	●	●		●	●
leg pull prone		●		●	●	●	●
lunge		●					
mermaid				●		●	●
Pilates push up		●	▼●	●	●		▼●
praying mantis		●		●	●	●	●
shoulder challenge				●	●	●	●
superman		●		●	●	●	●
swimming	●	●	●	●	●	●	●
teaser		●					
torpedo				●	●	●	●
waist twists in standing	●		●				

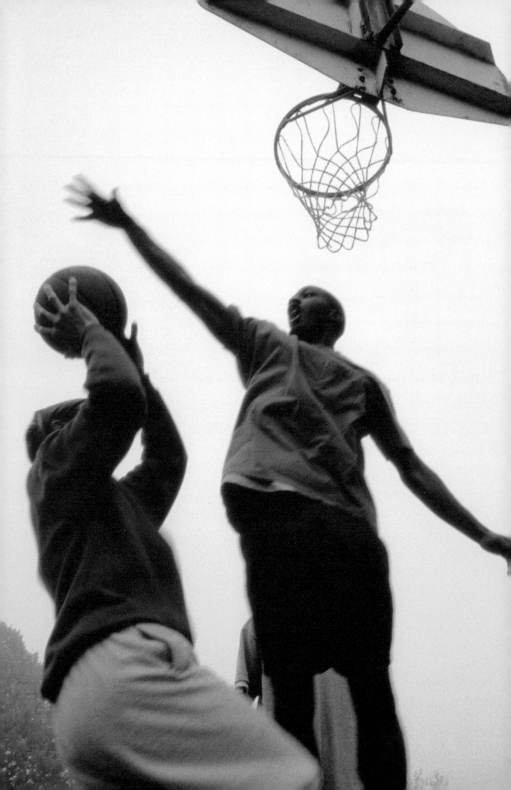

Basketball

In basketball and volleyball, rapid changes in direction, mistimed shots (causing contact with another player), and awkward landing can lead to sprained ankles and damaged knee ligaments.

The injuries that occur to those who play these sports are similar owing to the similar physical demands of the sports. All these can be prevented with good and regular use of Pilates exercises as shown in the chart at the end of the section.

INJURIES

ANTERIOR CRUCIATE
LIGAMENT

CALF MUSCLE STRAIN

PATELLAR TENDONITIS

ACHILLES TENDONITIS

ANKLE INVERSION INJURY

SHOULDER IMPINGEMENT

Common basketball injuries

Anterior cruciate ligament

The knee has four ligaments holding it in place: one at each side to stop the bones sliding sideways and two crossing over in the middle to stop the bones sliding forward and backward. It is the latter two, in the middle, that are called the cruciate ligaments: the posterior (the back) cruciate ligament and the anterior (the front) cruciate ligament. If these are damaged in any way they may cause knee pain. The main job of the anterior cruciate ligament in the knee is to passively stabilize the knee and supply lots of sensory information to the central nervous system.

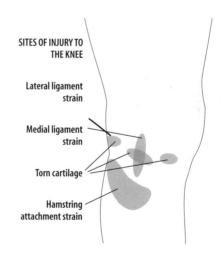

SITES OF INJURY TO
THE KNEE

Lateral ligament
strain

Medial ligament
strain

Torn cartilage

Hamstring
attachment strain

Causes

The ligament can be injured by twisting the knee or from an impact to the side of the knee—often on the outside.

Signs and symptoms

Sudden or gradual swelling of the knee. If the swelling takes place over a period of two hours, this can indicate a small amount of damage to the soft tissue.

The sensation of the knee separating or a "gapping" in the knee area when the injury occurs. This feeling occurs owing to a tear in the ligament.

Severe pain when the injury occurs. It's unlikely you'll be able to continue playing. The pain may dissipate quickly and you'll be able to move your knee forward, but any twisting movement will cause pain again. This is owing to the instability of the knee stabilizers.

Use the anterior draw test (see page 125) to determine the extent of the injury.

Treatment

IMMEDIATE

Control the swelling through the use of P.R.I.C.E (see page 9) on the knee area.

Ice will help reduce the amount of pain.

LONG-TERM

The extent of the overall injury is determined by the degree of damage to the ligament. Complete or near partial rupture may require repair or reconstruction, and will need to be assessed by a medical practitioner.

If the ligament has been stretched and not torn, indicated by the minimal amount of swelling and failure of the anterior draw test, then follow the treatment plan for knee ligaments on pages 123–7.

Rehabilitation

Build up the support of the quadriceps muscles.

Maintain a general level of fitness through aqua jogging and cycling or walking.

Follow the Pilates program at the end of this chapter to help improve your lower-limb balance, coordination, and endurance.

How to prevent

Make sure that you are fit enough to play. Don't use the game to improve your fitness levels.

Make sure you warm up completely before playing. Do not attempt to take a shot without warming up correctly.

Follow a comprehensive fitness routine. This should involve 8–12 exercises from the program at the end of this chapter.

Make sure you are wearing the correct footwear (see page 16).

Always wear shin pads.

Maintain strength in the trunk, pelvis, and abdominal muscles.

Proprioception—balance—is the secret to preventing injuries in the lower body. Follow your Pilates program completely and regularly.

Stop exercising or playing if you experience any pain.

Don't push yourself too hard. Stop if you feel tired.

Concentrate on exercises to improve your coordination skills and agility.

Calf muscle strain

The calf muscles consist of the gastrocnemius, which is the big muscle at the back of the lower leg, and the soleus muscle, which is a smaller muscle lower down in the leg and under the gastrocnemius. Either of these two muscles can be strained or torn.

A sudden sharp pain in the calf muscle followed by difficulty using it, is usually a give away for a calf strain. The most common place to get this injury is at the muscle/tendon junction of the gastrocnemius roughly halfway between the knee and the heel. Test for this by contracting the muscle against resistance with your legs straight. Pain is felt midway up the calf muscle.

Causes

Failing to warm up properly before a game.

Repetitive slapping down of foot while the knee is extended. Pain is usually felt immediately in the calf muscle.

Excessive lunging.

Suddenly ceasing sporting activity, such as running, without warming down correctly.

Signs and symptoms

Sudden sharp pain in the calf muscle.

Being unable to continue with activity.

Treatment

IMMEDIATE

Apply ice for ten minutes.

Undertake the P.R.I.C.E. recovery plan.

Reduce the amount of weight on the leg by using a crutch or by resting.

Use a heel raise in your shoe if you are unable to walk on the flat without experiencing sharp pain.

Maintain a range of motion exercises—but don't do any movements that stretch the muscle.

Flex the foot backward and forward (active dorsiflexion/plantar flexion) to test for pain.

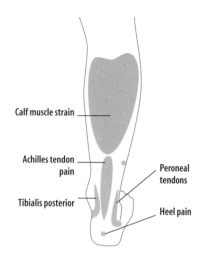

Calf muscle strain

Achilles tendon pain

Peroneal tendons

Tibialis posterior

Heel pain

LONG-TERM

Only resume exercising when pain has diminished or completely gone. Only enter into moderate activity when tolerable.

How to prevent

Warm up adequately for the game.

Follow the lengthening program for calf muscles at the end of this chapter.

Achilles tendonitis

Achilles tendonitis is an inflammation condition and is an overuse injury.

The Achilles tendon, the largest tendon in the body, connects the gastrocnemius and soleus muscles to the heel and transfers the force of their contractions to lift the heel.

Causes

Turning the foot over while running.

Straining the Achilles tendon while running or jumping.

Years of jumping and/or running during sports and training.

Increasing sporting activity without increasing physical fitness levels.

Change of training surface.

New or ill-fitting footwear.

Weakness in the calf.

Tight gastrocnemius.

Restricted dorsiflexion.

Excessive pronation of the ankle and foot, which causes the Achilles tendon to pull off-center, resulting in inflammation.

Signs and symptoms

Experiencing widespread and severe pain in the tendons.

Burning pain in the tendon.

Pain is felt in the whole tendon.

Pain occurs gradually.

Achilles tendon feels painful and stiff in the morning.

Achilles tendon is tender to squeeze between thumb and index finger. The area of inflammation will be indicated by the presence of pain when squeezed.

Treatment

IMMEDIATE

Avoid placing any impact on the foot.

Relative rest.

Include heel drops (page 207) in your warm up program.

Acute pain may resolve itself within 3 to 4 weeks.

LONG-TERM

Gradually build up strength within the calf muscles.

Concentrate on performing heel drops (see page 207) at a set speed on one leg. If you do not experience any pain, you

should have sufficient strength to begin training again.

Incorporate the Pilates program outlined at the end of this chapter into your workout routine.

How to prevent

Maintain length in the ankle dorsiflexion muscles (ankle pulled up toward you).

Maintain strength in the tendon, as indicated in the treatment program at the end of this chapter.

Ankle inversion injury

Ankle sprains are by far the most common injuries in sports. They are usually caused by the ankle rolling over and forcing the foot into dorsiflexion and inversion.

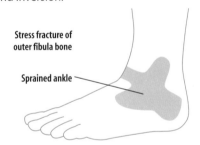

Stress fracture of outer fibula bone

Sprained ankle

Causes

Landing awkwardly from a jump.

Stepping or landing on your opponent's foot during a game.

Changing direction suddenly.

Sudden deceleration during run.

Running on an uneven surface.

Weak peronal (ankle) muscles.

Tight Achilles tendon.

Previous ankle injury.

Signs and symptoms

Being able to pinpoint the exact location and feeling of the injury.

Hearing a popping sound.

Feeling a tearing sensation, followed by a sharp pain.

Finding the area painful to touch.

Being unable to walk without feeling pain in the area.

Swelling or bruising on the side of the foot.

Treatment

IMMEDIATE

Control pain and swelling through the following procedures:

P.R.I.C.E.

Bear weight only when it is tolerable.

Try to write the alphabet in the air with your foot to test the range of pain-free motion.

LONG-TERM

Achieve a good sense of balance with the ankle.

Build strength around the ankle joint.

Be sensitive to pain when you feel it.

How to prevent

Maintain good strength and coordination around the ankle joint.

Follow the exercise program at the end of this chapter to improve your performance and prevent ankle injury.

Shoulder impingement

Injuries around the shoulder occur while playing owing to three main reasons:

1. Excessive movement of the shoulder joint in the capsule of the joint.

2. There is mechanical obstruction of the rotator cuff tendons under the anterior inferior of the acromion and associated loss of space in the subacromial area.

3. Muscle imbalance owing to changes of muscle length and strength in the muscles around the shoulder and shoulder blade.

Causes

Imbalance of muscles around the shoulder owing to changes in the muscles of the rotator cuff.

Weakness of the muscle at the back of the shoulder joint.

Tightness with internal rotation of the shoulder joint owing to shortening of the external rotator muscles (infraspinatus).

Too much external rotation of the actual shoulder joint.

Identify the painful phase of the stroke to help determine the structures involved.

Pilates exercises to improve performance and prevent further injury

▮ Lengthen
▼ Balance
● Strengthen

	Anterior cruciate ligament	Calf muscle strain	Achilles tendonitis	Ankle inversion injury	Shoulder impingement
CORE EXERCISES					
curl up	●	●	●	●	●
diamond press					●
floating arms					●
four point challenge	●			▼	▼
hip opening	●	●	●	●	
pelvic stability	●	●	●	●	
neutral spine	●	●			
static standing balance	▼	▼	▼	▼	
FOUNDATION EXERCISES					
arm circles				●	▮●
arm opening				▮	▮▼
big squeeze		●			
dart		▼		▮	▮▼●
hamstring lengthening	▮	▮		▮●	
long sitting stretch		▮	▮●	●	●
mid-back stretch					▮●
roll downs		▮	●	▮●	●
shoulder external rotation					●
shoulder push away					●
shoulder rowing					●
shoulder rotation control					●
shoulder internal rotation					●
side reach		●			●
single knee kicks	▮●			▮●	
spinal curls			▮●	●	
standing squat	●	●	●	●	
star					●
T-band balance	▼	▼	▼	▼	
wall slides		●	●	●	

	Anterior cruciate ligament	Calf muscle strain	Achilles tendonitis	Ankle inversion injury	Shoulder impingement
PERFORMANCE PILATES					
bridging	●	●	●	●	
double leg stretch		●			▼●
eccentric hamstrings	●	●			
hundred		●	●		●
knee circles	▮●	▮			
lean forward bending		●	●	●	
leg pull back	●				
leg pull prone	●	●			●
lunge		●	●	●	
mermaid					●
open leg rocker	▮●	●			
Pilates push up					▼●
praying mantis	●				●
roll up		▮			
rolling like a ball			▮		
scissors	●	●	●		
shoulder challenge					●
side kick series		●		●	
side rolls	●	▮			
single leg stretch	●	●	▮●	●	
sitting knee folds	●				
superman					●
swimming	▮●	●	●		●
teaser		●			
tennis ball raises	●	▮●	●	●	
torpedo	●	●	●		●
wrist strengthening					●▮

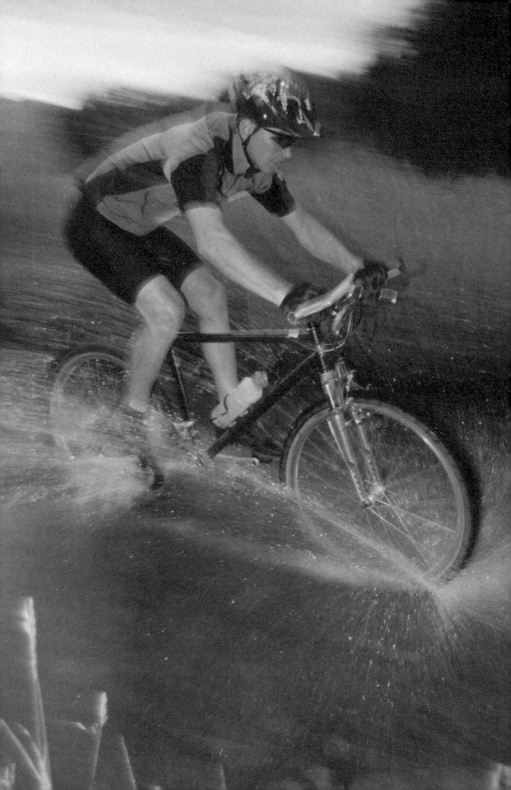

Cycling

Injuries caused during cycling can occur in one of two ways: either because of the fit of the bike itself or of how the cyclist fits on the bike. If the bike doesn't fit the rider, injuries such as neck strain and back pain can occur. Injuries such as strains or leg pain occur mainly because of overuse, overtraining, or not warming up or down sufficiently.

Common cycling injuries

Neck strain

A strain is a tear in a muscle or tendon. Your neck is surrounded by small muscles, which run close to the vertebrae, and larger muscles, which are the neck muscles that you see. Neck strains often occur when the head and neck are held in an uncomfortable position for a long period of time.

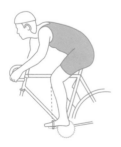

Poor neck position can lead to neck strain.

Causes

Dropping the head due to the position of the handlebars.

Poking your chin out when riding.

Muscle fatigue in arms and shoulders.

Signs and symptoms

Pain or stiffness in the nape of the neck.

Muscle strain or dull ache in the upper shoulder area.

Treatment
IMMEDIATE

Stretch your shoulders (trapezius muscles) as regularly as possible.

LONG-TERM

Maintain good muscle position in the neck muscles.

How to prevent

Stretch your trapezius muscles.

Strengthen your deep neck flexors.

Change your bike for one that fits you correctly.

Raise your handlebars to allow you to sit upright.

Wear a lighter helmet.

Tilt your neck and lengthen through the thoracic spine to achieve the correct long-neck position.

Iliotibial band syndrome

Iliotibial band syndrome is one of the leading causes of lateral knee pain in cyclists. The iliotibial band is a superficial thickening of tissue on the outside of the thigh, extending from the outside of the pelvis, over the hip and knee, and inserting just below the knee. The band is crucial to stabilizing the knee when pedaling.

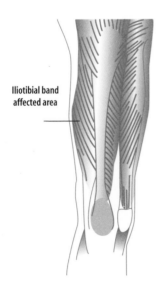

Iliotibial band affected area

Causes

Cycling too much, too soon after injury, without sufficient fitness.

A tight iliotibial tract which is brought on by "bowing" knees (turning inward) and/or foot pronation or flat feet (feet turning inward), which can all lead to the lower limb turning inward.

A fall on to the hip.

Signs and symptoms

Pain is localized in the greater trochanter on the lateral aspect of the hip (this pain is often experienced by long-distance cyclists).

Inflammation is aggravated by hip movements (for example, when running, or getting out of the car).

There is a catching or snapping of the bursa (the fluid-filled sac in this area) across the greater trochanter.

There is pain and tenderness over the trochanter. Pain increases with any weight-bearing movement.

See a medical professional to make an accurate diagnosis. This injury can sometimes be a stress fracture along the neck of the femur or referred pain from the spine and/or the sacroiliac joint.

Treatment

IMMEDIATE

Stretch out the iliotibial band.

Take a rest from cycling until pain disappears.

Cycle for shorter distances.

Avoid cycling in a high gear.

Take anti-inflammatory tablets (as directed) to reduce pain.

Iliotibial band syndrome

This injury has the same symptoms as tronchanteric gluteal pain but the pain is caused by the inflammation of the actual iliotibial band because it is tight. There is also friction of the band on the greater trochanter (the far point of the hip joint).

Differences between Iliotibial band syndrome and tronchanteric gluteal pain:

Cycling in a high gear is painful.

Pain is felt when cycling on uneven banks.

Pain is localized to the greater trochanter on the lateral aspect of the hip (this pain is often experienced by long-distance runners).

The inflammation is aggravated by certain hip movements such as cycling or getting out of the car.

There is a catching or snapping of the bursa (the fluid-filled sac in this area) across the greater trochanter.

Use taping on the gluteal area if the area is causing irritation.

Regularly follow the stretching and strengthening exercises at the end of this chapter. This will minimize symptoms in about a week. If you practice these exercises less frequently, it may take up to six weeks to improve.

LONG-TERM

When you return to regular training, avoid going over steep cambers on the road. Keep to flat surfaces and build up your distance on the flat.

Alter your training schedule if the pain is only present when you are training.

Try reducing your cycling distance by half if you are still experiencing problems.

OBER'S TEST

Allow the top, straight leg to drop down below the table level.

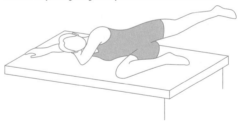

Tightness in the iliotibial band is indicated if the top leg is unable to reach this position.

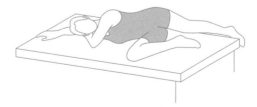

Prevention

Maintain the ratio between the length and strength of the muscles around the hip, particularly the gluteus medius and deep hip rotators by undertaking the program outlined at the end of this chapter.

Adjust the seat height and/or change the frame size of your bike.

Cycling knee pain

This common condition for cyclists is a result of softening and changes to the under-surface of the kneecap.

Diagram of affected area: sites of pain.

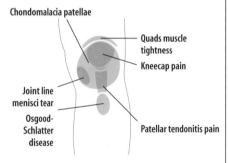

Chondomalacia patellae

Quads muscle tightness

Kneecap pain

Joint line menisci tear

Osgood-Schlatter disease

Patellar tendonitis pain

Causes

Incorrect frame size.

Seat is too high.

Incorrect cycling technique or too much cycling can place repetitive strain on the knee.

Excessive pronation of the foot and use of the quadriceps muscle in a bent-knee position.

Signs and symptoms

Poorly defined pain can vary from a dull ache to sharp pain depending on activity.

Pain is aggravated by walking down stairs or down a slope.

Pain can occur during prolonged sitting.

When standing after prolonged sitting, the knee locks, then gives way.

High repetitive stress in the inside of the knee (anterior). Incorrect alignment of the outside of the knee.

Treatment
IMMEDIATE

Apply ice for 10 minutes or until the area is numb.

LONG-TERM

Change the height of the cycle seat to decrease the amount of bend in the knee. If the seat is higher, less stress will be placed on the knee.

Change your cycling route and ride on flatter terrain.

Slowly increase the intensity and duration of your training periods.

Hamstring strain

This is the most common injury suffered by athletes. The hamstring is actually a group of three muscles that help to straighten (extend) the leg at the hip and bend (flex) the leg at the knee. The pull felt during injury is a strain or tear in the muscles or tendons.

Causes
ACUTE STRAIN

For cyclists, acute hamstring injury can be

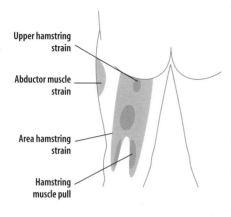

Upper hamstring strain

Abductor muscle strain

Area hamstring strain

Hamstring muscle pull

Diagram of affected area: sites of pain.

a result of increased intensity in cycling. Contributing factors are:

Failure to stretch before training.

Fatigue. Don't push your body when it is feeling the strain of training.

Training when you have an existing injury which has not been assessed.

Making the muscle weak by placing it under tension.

Tight neurological tissue as a result of restricted movement in the lumbar spine. If you do suffer from tightness in this area, you will need a detailed assessment from a medical practitioner.

CHRONIC STRAIN

Inadequate hamstring length indicated by tightness of the muscle.

Inadequate strength and flexibility in the hip rotator.

Increasing mileage too dramatically or changing cycling style.

Signs and symptoms

ACUTE

Increased inflexibility of the hamstrings.

Localized tenderness in the muscle.

Bruising at the back of the knee owing to muscle fibers tearing and bleeding.

Pain on bending to touch the toes.

CHRONIC

Soreness where the tissue has not completely healed, which indicates loss of elasticity within the muscle.

Treatment

IMMEDIATE

Place an ice pack on the affected muscle for ten minutes or until the area is numb.

Gently contract and relax the muscle.

Tape the muscle to prevent any over-pull on the fibres.

Take anti-inflammatory tablets to reduce pain and swelling.

LONG-TERM

Start training again slowly to test for pain.

See the exercises listed at the end of this chapter.

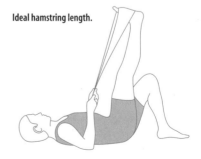

Ideal hamstring length.

Achilles tendonitis

The Achilles tendon, the largest tendon in the body, connects the gastrocnemius and soleus muscles to the heel bone. It transfers the force of contractions to lift the heel. Achilles tendonitis is an inflammation condition due to overuse.

Diagram of affected area: sites of pain.

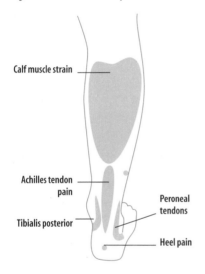

Calf muscle strain

Achilles tendon pain

Tibialis posterior

Peroneal tendons

Heel pain

Cause

Training on irregular surfaces.

Incorrect use of equipment.

Direct trauma to the Achilles (such as a blow or deep cut).

Sudden increase in mileage.

An intense training session.

Sudden increase in intensity.

Hill training.

Failure to warm up.

Recommencing training after a period of inactivity.

Sudden switch to cycling from other activities.

Stiff mid-foot.

Inadequate calf flexibility.

Signs and symptoms

Severe or widespread tendon pain.

Burning pain in the tendon.

Pain enveloping the entire tendon.

Gradual onset of the pain.

Pain/stiffness in the morning.

Achilles tendon is tender to squeeze between thumb and index finger. The area of inflammation will be indicated by the presence of pain when squeezed.

Treatment

IMMEDIATE

Avoid placing any impact on your foot.

Relative rest.

Acute pain may resolve itself within three to four weeks. Easily becomes chronic.

Include heel drops (page 207) in your warm-up program.

LONG-TERM

Gradually build up strength.

Concentrate on performing heel drops at a set speed on one leg. If you do not experience pain, you should have sufficient strength to begin training.

Incorporate the Pilates program at the end of this chapter into your routine.

Prevention

Maintain length in the ankle dorsiflexion muscles (ankle pulled up toward you).

Maintain strength in tendon, as indicated in the treatment program.

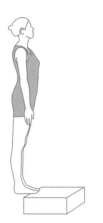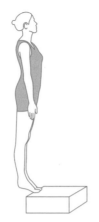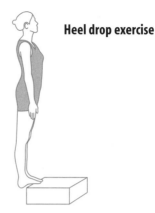

Heel drop exercise

Including heel drops in your warm up program can help prevent injuries to the Achilles tendon.

Remember the causes of injury and work to prevent the initial trigger.

Loosen the toe clips.

Adjust the seat height up or down to suit you.

Change foot position.

Lower the gear as you train.

Adjust pedaling techniques while cycling. Experiment with the gears to find one which doesn't place strain or cause pain to the Achilles tendon. Remain in this gear for your training sessions.

How to choose the correct bike for you

• You should be able to stand over your bike and have 1–3 inches (2–8cm) clearance over the bar. When sitting on the bike, with your feet on the ground, you should have a slight bend to your knee .

• Make sure you're balanced. About 40 percent of your body weight should be placed on the front half of the bike (handlebars) and 60 percent on the rear half of the bike.

• Bikes with shock absorbers will give a smoother ride and be easier on your bottom.

• The ideal recreational bike should have a suspension seat and wide tyres. A recumbent bike features a laid-back seating position, which provides great back support.

• There are different types of bike seats for men and women. Using the right type of seat reduces the strain on pressure points and makes for a more comfortable ride.

Pilates exercises to improve performance and prevent further injury

▮ Lengthen
▼ Balance
● Strengthen

	Neck strain	Cycling knee	Iliotibial band syndrome	Hamstring muscle strain	Achilles tendonitis
CORE EXERCISES					
curl up	●			●	●
diamond press	●	▮			
floating arms	●				
four point challenge	▼	▼	▼		
hip opening			●	●	●
imprinting		●			
pelvic stability				●	●
static standing balance			▼		
FOUNDATION EXERCISES					
arm opening	●				
big squeeze				●	
dart	●			●	
long sitting stretch		▮			●
mid-back stretch	●				
neck rolls	●				
roll downs	▮				▮
shoulder rotation control	●				
side reach	●	●		●	
single knee kicks			●	●	
spinal curls		▮		●	▮●
standing squat			●	●	●
star	●				
T-band balance			▼		▼
threading the needle	●				
wall slides	▮		●	●	▮●
windows	●				

PERFORMANCE PILATES	Neck strain	Cycling knee	Iliotibial band syndrome	Hamstring muscle strain	Achilles tendonitis
bridging			●	●	●
double leg stretch	●	●		●	
heel drop					●
hundred	●	●		●	●
leg pull back	●				
leg pull prone	●				
lunge					●
oblique curl up		●			
open leg rocker					●
Pilates push up	●				
praying mantis	●		●	●	
roll up				●	
rolling like a ball					▮
scissors					▮ ●
side kick series			●	●	●
side rolls				●	
single leg stretch	●				▮ ●
sitting knee folds				●	●
swimming	●	●	●	●	●
teaser	●				
tennis ball raises			●		●
torpedo			●	●	●

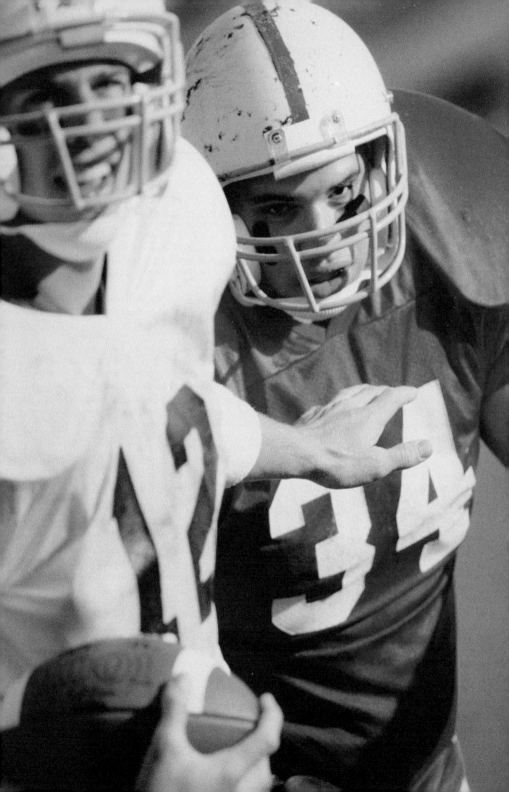

Football

Football is an extremely high-contact sport. Injuries tend to occur when players compete physically for the ball, and to prevent the opposing team from touching it, posing considerable risk to the neck and shoulders as well as causing minor contusions or lacerations. The most common football injuries are sprains, particularly ligament sprains, and strains to muscles or tendons.

Common football injuries

Shoulder dislocation

A shoulder dislocation is when the top part of the arm bone (humeral head) slips out of its socket (glenoid cavity). Forward (anterior) dislocations are most common. When this occurs the anterior inferior labrum (a piece of cartilage that stabilizes the shoulder) frequently is torn. Shoulder dislocations can also occur backward (posterior) and downward (inferior).

Causes

Falling is the most common cause of a new shoulder dislocation. It occurs when the arm is forcibly moved into an awkward position during a fall. If a dislocation or partial dislocation (known as a subluxation) occurs with only a minor amount of force, recurrent injury then instability may be considered.

Signs and symptoms

Loss of active range of movement in the shoulder joint in most directions.

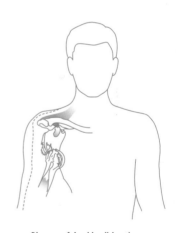

Diagram of shoulder dislocation

A feeling that the joint has "popped out'"

Loss of normal profile or appearance in the shoulder region.

Treatment

IMMEDIATE

Seek medical attention.

Place the arm in a sling for approximately ten days, making sure the elbow does not get stiff and the neck maintains a normal range of motion.

Practice isometric exercises using the rotator cuff muscles, while in a neutral joint position to help your range of flexibility.

Seek expert advice about the ideal rehabilitation program in order to prevent a recurrence of the injury.

N.B. If this is the first time you have dislocated your shoulder, the relocation may occur without assistance.

LONG-TERM

Strengthen the muscle, taking at least six to twelve weeks to do so.

Don't expect full strength to return for six months or more.

Check the range of movement in the muscle around the shoulder joint in order to determine the presence of any muscle imbalances.

Respect the pain you are experiencing. You may have to limit how often you play until your shoulder heals.

How to prevent

Maintain a good strength and coordination in the shoulder and rotator cuff area (see page 33).

Hamstring strain

This is the most common injury suffered by football players and athletes in general. The hamstring is actually a group of three muscles that help to straighten (extend) the leg at the hip and bend (flex) the leg at the knee. The pull felt during an injury is a strain or tear in the muscles or tendons.

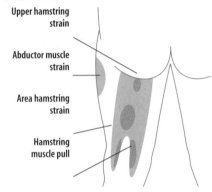

Upper hamstring strain

Abductor muscle strain

Area hamstring strain

Hamstring muscle pull

Hamstring muscles strain: sites of pain.

Causes

ACUTE STRAIN

Acute hamstring injury can occur when a football player increases sprinting intensity. Contributing factors are:

Cold weather. Make sure you stretch before playing to warm up your muscles.

Fatigue. Don't push your body when it is feeling the strain of training.

Playing when you have a preexisting injury in the hamstring.

Making the muscle weak by placing it under tension. This tends to happen when football players sprint or slip.

Tight neurological tissue as a result of restricted movement in the lumbar spine.

If you do suffer from tightness in this area, you will need a detailed assessment from a medical practitioner.

CHRONIC STRAIN

Inadequate hamstring length indicated by tightness of the muscle.

Inadequate strength and flexibility in the hip rotator.

Signs and symptoms

ACUTE

Increased inflexibility of the hamstrings.

Localized tenderness in the muscle.

Bruising at the back of the knee owing to muscle fibers tearing and bleeding.

Pain on bending to touch the toes.

CHRONIC

Soreness where the tissue has not completely healed, which indicates loss of elasticity within the muscle.

Treatment

IMMEDIATE

Place an ice pack on the affected muscle for ten minutes or until the area is numb.

Gently contract and relax the muscle.

Tape the muscle to prevent any overpull on the fibers.

Take anti-inflammatory tablets to reduce pain and swelling.

LONG-TERM

Start training again slowly to test for pain.

See the exercises listed at the end of this chapter.

Medial ligament strain

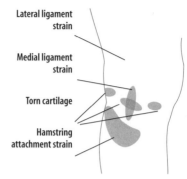

Lateral ligament strain

Medial ligament strain

Torn cartilage

Hamstring attachment strain

Sites of potential knee injury.

Causes

This strain can occur when the player goes in for a block tackle forcing or twisting the knee. The knee may be twisted if the foot is fixed firmly on the ground (possibly owing to the cleats of the shoe).

Signs and symptoms

Pain on the inside of the knee. The amount of pain will determine the degree of injury present.

Swelling in the knee.

Tenderness along the length of the ligament.

Pain when running, particularly when attempting a sudden change in direction.

Discomfort when using the inside of the foot to kick the ball.

Treatment

IMMEDIATE

P.R.I.C.E. Control swelling with the application of ice, for ten minutes or until the area is numb.

Mc Murray test: Lie down and bend your injured knee. Ask a partner to put one hand over your knee, while supporting your heel with the other hand. Pulling up on your heel, they should gently turn your knee outward and straighten your leg (keeping your knee turned out). Bend your leg again and this time rotate the knee inward by pressing around the heel, and then straighten the leg. Pain in achieving a straight leg indicates a positive result.

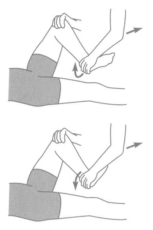

Meniscus tear

There are two menisci in your knee which rest between the thigh bone (femur) and shin bone (tibia). One meniscus rests on the medial tibial plateau; this is the medial meniscus. The other meniscus rests on the lateral tibial plateau—the lateral meniscus. The meniscus' main function is to distribute the weight evenly in the leg, to prevent any damage to the knee joint.

The most common traumatic meniscus tear occurs when the knee joint is bent (flexed) and the knee is then twisted. It is not uncommon for the meniscus tear to occur along with injuries to the anterior cruciate ligament and the medial collateral ligament. When all three occur together they are known as the "unhappy triad'", which may happen in sports such as football when the player is hit on the outside of the knee.

Protect the ligament from further damage: wear a brace or tape the knee.

LONG-TERM

Reduce or minimize the swelling by applying ice for ten minutes, or until the area is numb. Apply every two hours.

Build up the support of the quadriceps.

Maintain a general level of fitness, through aqua jogging, or cycling, as long as the pain is minimal.

Participate in activities that build up your lower-limb balance and coordination of movement.

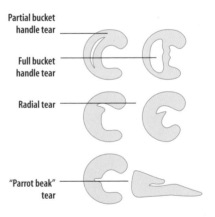

Partial bucket handle tear

Full bucket handle tear

Radial tear

"Parrot beak" tear

Types of meniscus tears

Causes

Twisting the knee while the foot is anchored to the ground.

Progressive wear on the whole joint (often found in people over 40).

Signs and symptoms

Swelling proportional to activity.

Pain on rotation or flexion.

Pain on joint line.

Feeling of weakness and insecurity in the legs, or the knee actually giving way.

Locking sensation in the knee.

Generalized ache in the knee.

Positive McMurray test (see left).

Treatment
CONSERVATIVE

Symptoms develop over 24 hours.

There is minimal swelling.

There is full range of movement, with pain only at end of range.

Pain during McMurray test in the inner range of flexion.

Surgery may be required if:

Injury is due to severe twisting motion.

Player is unable to continue.

Knee clicks during McMurray test.

Tear associated with anterior cruciate ligament.

Little improvement after three weeks of ongoing treatment.

Treatment
IMMEDIATE

Control swelling through P.R.I.C.E.

Maintain an active range of motion.

Maintain a contraction of the quadriceps for the count of three, then release.

LONG-TERM

Keep swelling to a minimum by applying ice regularly after exercise if pain continues.

Continue stretching to maintain a full range of movement.

Follow the Pilates program at the end of this chapter.

How to prevent

Train all-year round to ensure you are fit enough for the football season. This will help prevent muscle injuries.

Strengthen the particular muscles used during a game: neck, abdominals, and the trunk.

Always warm up before starting a game.

Follow the Pilates flexibility program at the end of this chapter.

Strained calf muscles

The calf muscles consist of the gastrocnemius, which is the big muscle at the back of the lower leg and the soleus muscle, which is a smaller muscle lower down in the leg and under the gastrocnemius. Either of these two muscles can be strained or torn. A sudden sharp pain in the calf muscle followed by difficulty using it usually indicates calf strain. The most common place to get this injury is roughly halfway between the knee and the heel. You can test for this by contracting the muscle against resistance with the legs straight. Pain is felt midway up the calf muscle.

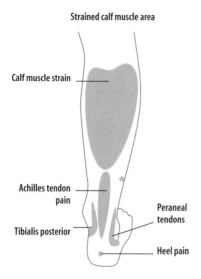

Strained calf muscle area

Calf muscle strain

Achilles tendon pain

Peraneal tendons

Tibialis posterior

Heel pain

Reduce the amount of weight on the leg by using a crutch or resting.

Use a heel raise in your shoe if you are unable to walk on a flat surface without experiencing sharp pain.

Maintain a range of motion exercises— but do not perform any movements that stretch the calf muscle.

Flex the foot backward and forward (active dorsiflexion/plantar flexion) to test for pain.

LONG-TERM

Resume exercising when pain has completely gone. Enter into moderate activity only when tolerable.

How to prevent

Warm up adequately for the game.

Follow the lengthening program for calf muscles at the end of this chapter.

Ankle inversion injury

Causes

Landing awkwardly from a jump.

Stepping or landing on your opponent's foot during the game.

Changing direction suddenly or a sudden deceleration during run.

Running on an uneven surface.

Weak peroneal muscles.

Tight Achilles tendon.

Existing ankle injury.

Signs and symptoms

You are able to describe the actual mechanism of injury.

Causes

Failing to warm up properly before training or a game.

Repetitive slapping down of foot while the knee is extended. Pain is usually immediately felt in the calf muscle.

Excessive lunging when not warmed up.

Suddenly ceasing activity, such as stopping running, without warming down correctly.

Signs and symptoms

Sudden sharp pain in the calf muscle.

Being unable to continue with activity.

Treatment

IMMEDIATE

Undertake the P.R.I.C.E recovery plan. Apply the ice for ten minutes immediately after feeling the pain.

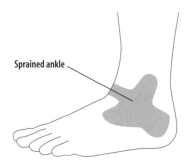

Sprained ankle

Stress fracture of the out fibula bone.

The ankle hurts to touch, even at rest.
You are unable to walk without pain.
Swelling and bruising on side of the foot.

What sort of sprain do you have?

MILD SPRAIN
You do not limp when walking.

MODERATE SPRAIN
There is a noticeable limp when walking.
You cannot raise up on your toes or hop on your injured ankle.

SEVERE SPRAIN
It is painful to place weight on the injured foot.
You find it difficult to walk without any assistance.

Treatment

IMMEDIATE
Control pain and swelling through the following procedure:
P.R.I.C.E.

Bear weight on the ankle only when it is tolerable.
Write the alphabet in the air with your foot to test range of pain-free motion.

LONG-TERM
Achieve a good sense of balance with the ankle (joint proprioception).
Build strength around the ankle joint.
Be sensitive to pain when you feel it.
Respect the pain during sport.

Prevention
Maintain good strength and coordination around the ankle joint.
Follow the exercise program at the end of this chapter to improve your performance and prevent further ankle injury.

Pilates exercises to improve performance and prevent further injury

I Lengthen
▼ Balance
● Strengthen

	Ankle inversion injury	Medial ligament strain	Meniscus tear	Shoulder dislocation	Hamstring strain	Calf muscle strain
Core exercises						
curl up		●	●	●	●	
diamond press				●		
floating arms				●		
four point challenge				▼	I	▼
hip opening	●	●	●		●	
pelvic stability	●	●	●		●	●
static standing balance		▼	▼			▼
Foundation exercises						
arm circles				●		
arm opening				I		
big squeeze				●		
dart				I●	●	
hamstring lengthening	●	I				
long sitting stretch	●	●	●	●		
mid-back stretch				●		
roll downs	I●			●		I
shoulder external rotation				●		
shoulder internal rotation				●		
shoulder push away				●		
shoulder rowing				●		
side reach				●	●	
single knee kicks	I●	I●	I		I●	●
spinal curls	●	●			●	
standing squat	●	●	●		●	
star		●		●		
T-band balance		▼	▼		▼	▼
wall slides	I●		●		●	I●

Performance Pilates	Ankle inversion injury	Medial ligament strain	Meniscus tear	Shoulder dislocation	Hamstring strain	Calf muscle strain
bridging	●	●	●		●	
double leg stretch				▮●	●	
eccentric hamstrings		●				
hundred				●	●	●
knee/leg circles		▮●				
lean forward bending	●					
leg pull back		●				
leg pull prone		●		●		
lunge	●					
mermaid				●		
open leg rocker		▮●	●			
Pilates push up				▼●		
praying mantis		●		●	●	
roll up					●	●
rolling like a ball			●			
scissors		●				
shoulder challenge				●		
side kick series	▮●		●		●	
side rolls		●			●	
single leg stretch	▮●	●				●
sitting knee folds		●			●	
superman				●		
swimming	▮	▮●	●	●	●	●
tennis ball raises	▮●	●	●			●
torpedo		●		●	●	

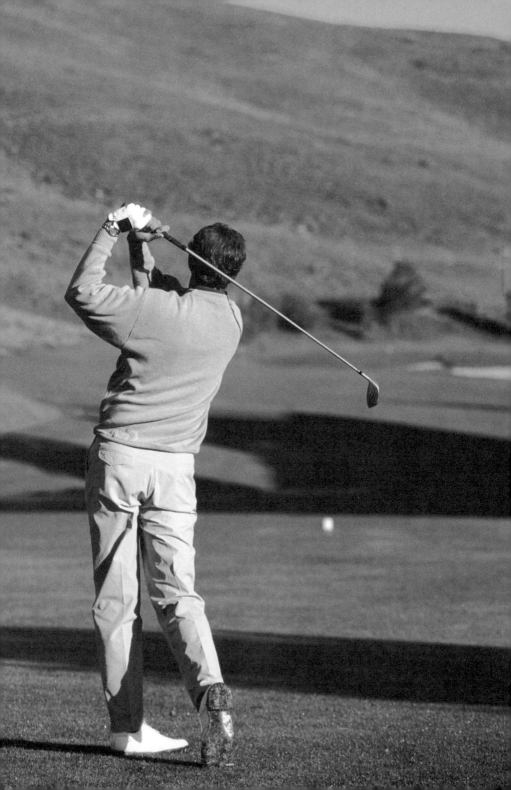

Golf

Playing golf may look like a relatively slow-moving activity, but it actually places a lot of strain on the body. Picking up the golf bag, swinging a golf club, constantly twisting the upper torso, and bending to pick up golf balls are all responsible for causing pain in the golfer's back, shoulders, and wrists. In this section we look at the pains associated with an incorrect golf swing and how to improve your swing techniques to prevent further injury.

INJURIES
___

LOW BACK PAIN

GOLFER'S SHOULDER

GOLFER'S ELBOW
___

Common golfing injuries

Low back pain

During a golf swing, the lumbar spine is subjected to forces caused by side bending, forward and backward shearing, compression, and rotation.

If you attempt to lift your leg to 90 degrees while experiencing back pain you will feel a restriction in the hip and lower back area and the pain will usually limit your movement to a range of only 60 degrees.

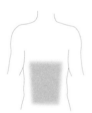

Causes

Existing occupational or domestic injuries often as a result of prolonged periods of sitting, as well as gardening and poor lifting techniques.

Prolonged bending during golf practice.

Extended periods of golf practice.

Weakness in the muscle groups needed in golf practice: abdominals, gluteals, and hamstrings.

Excessive forceful movement during a golf swing.

Constant flexing and straightening of your lower back muscles while playing.

Picking up golf balls without bending at the knees.

Prolonged periods of standing, especially if play is slow.

Incorrectly lifting, assembling and handling your golf buggy and bag.

Repeated twisting during the back swing and the follow through.

Failure to stretch before, during, and after golf game.

Treatment

IMMEDIATE

Adjust golf swing (see page 65 for instructions on correct golf swing).

Minimize the difference between shoulder rotation and hip rotation during the golf swing.

Keep your spine perpendicular to the ground when following through on a shot to minimize the twist and strain to the spine.

LONG-TERM

Make sure you complete your warm up stretches before playing. Try the following:

Place your golf club behind your back (arms fully extended) and rotate your trunk to warm up the lower back muscles.

Hold the golf club at shoulder height in front of you (parallel to the ground). Rotate your trunk.

How to prevent

Warm up before playing golf.

Make sure your swing is correct.

Strengthen key muscles: abdominals, obliques, gluteals, and trunk extensor muscles (see page 163).

Reduce any excessive forceful movements during "follow-through" stage of the swing.

Don't pick up the golf balls without bending your knees.

Always return to your normal posture after taking your shot.

Don't twist too much during the back swing and always follow through.

Warm up

Warm up for at least 30 minutes before playing a game.

Undertake specific golf stretching and swinging exercises.

Technique training

If you wish to improve your performance, take the time to enroll in professional lessons. Ask at your local golf club for information.

Golfer's shoulder

Injuries that can occur:

Rotator cuff strain (supraspinatus tendonitis).

Painful arc.

Impingement.

Rotator cuff area

Broken collarbone
Shoulder separation
Dislocation
Shoulder impingement
Rotator cuff
Biceps tendonitis

Causes

Golfing shoulder is usually caused by overuse of the shoulder area, rather than any specific component of the swing itself. During the golf swing, the leading shoulder is subject to an extreme range of motion, from internal rotation and adduction across the body at the top of the back swing to abduction and external rotation at the end of the follow-through.

If the amount of rotation in the spine is limited, then the shoulder will attempt to compensate for the limitation.

Continual repetition of a movement.

Underlying pathology such as arthritis.

Correct golf swing

Back swing
Associated problems:
Limitation in shoulder rotation and neck rotation
Tightness in hamstrings
Limited side bend
Pilates exercises
Threading the needle (page 200)
Spinal curls (page 196)
Side reach (page 194)

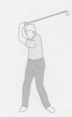

Downswing
Associated problems:
Limitation in the thoracic/spinal rotation
Tightness in hamstrings
Pilates exercises
Threading the needle (page 200)
Arm opening (page 180)

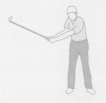

Acceleration ball strike
Associated problems:
Tightness in shoulder rotators,
particularly externally
Pilates exercises
Shoulder rotation control (page 192)
Dart (page 183)

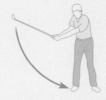

Follow-through
Associated problems:
Tight external shoulder rotation
Pilates exercises
Shoulder rotation (page 189–190)
Oblique curl up (page 215)
Waist twists in standing (page 232)
Threading the needle (page 200)
Side reach (page 194)

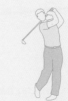

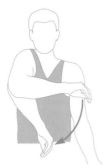

Test for anterior impingement of a rotator cuff muscle.

Failure to stretch before, during and after.

Poor technique in a golf swing.

The golf shaft is too rigid.

Vibrational shock through the arm if the club head hits the ground.

Strain on the joints from carrying a heavy golf bag.

Falling onto an outstretched hand.

Signs and symptoms

The location of the pain in the shoulder area can help in the diagnosis.

At the top of the back swing, pain in the front aspect of the lead shoulder is usually due to degenerative changes in the acromioclavicular joint or due to impingement.

Pain in the back is due to shoulder capsule tightness.

During follow-through, posterior pain in the lead shoulder is due to impingement.

Pinpointing the pain

Pain in the shoulder blades

Muscle weakness may be present around the shoulder blade. This can be indicated by the shoulder blade sticking out from the trunk on its inside border when the hand is placed behind the back.

Pain and weakness in the shoulder

Weakness in the shoulder external rotators (teres minor, infraspinatus), is indicated by the inability to turn the upper arm outward and inward. If you cannot put your hand behind your head without any discomfort, this may indicate weakness.

Treatment

IMMEDIATE

Application of P.R.I.C.E.

Reduce the stress on the acromio-clavicular joint by shortening the backswing. End the backswing at an imaginary one o'clock instead of three o'clock.

Work on your swing with a professional, in order to improve the mechanics.

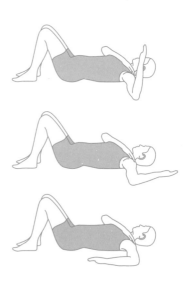

Diagram of internal rotation.

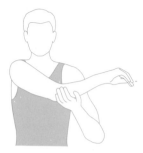

Posterior capsule stretch.

LONG-TERM

Strengthen the decelerators/scapular stabilizers muscles (rhomboids, serratus anterior).

How to prevent

See shoulder rotation control.

Aim to achieve a range of internal rotation greater than 80 degrees while in a 90-degree abducted position.

Undertake Pilates program as per chart at the end of the chapter.

Golfer's elbow

If there is pain in the inside of the elbow (medial elbow pain) this can indicate the presence of golfer's elbow. If the pain is on the outside (lateral elbow pain) it is likely to indicate the presence of tennis elbow.

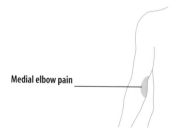

Medial elbow pain

The incidence of golfer's elbow increases with age and the number of rounds played. Playing more than two or three rounds per week can increase the probability of golfer's elbow.

Causes

Gripping the club too hard places increased shock on the elbow.

Overemphasizing the wrist release on contact with the ball.

Poor swing technique.

Swinging the club too forcefully.

Women tend to have an increased angle of the elbow compared to men.

Treatment

IMMEDIATE

Place ice on the local area for ten minutes or until the area is numb.

Take anti-inflammatory tablets to reduce the inflammation.

Modify painful activities for two weeks.

Have a golf professional assess your golfing technique.

LONG TERM

Have an assessment by a chartered physiotherapist. They will review the possible involvement of your cervical spine and restriction to the movement of your neural tissue that may be referring pain into the elbow area.

Improve your swing technique.

Changing your equipment may help reduce the vibration transmitted to your wrist and forearm.

Reduce the amount of rounds of golf you play.

Improve your conditioning technique.

Warm-up regime

1. When hitting balls on a driving range, start with short pitch shots (using short, low-intensity swing), before graduating to a full-swing lofted club.
2. Increase loft, length of swing, and number of shots. This allows the body to cope with the effort and strain placed on your body.
3. Practice putting before going onto the course to help postural alignment.

Flexibility tests

1. Test for: Neck rotation

While sitting upright in a chair, keep your shoulder and mid-back against the chair, turn your head to the right and the left, while keeping your chin parallel to the floor. Take care not to dip your head back in order to increase the anticipated range.

Ideal range: 70-90 degree rotation.

Influence on your golf game: Restricted neck rotation may lead you to take your eyes off the ball during the back swing.

Pilates exercises: Neck rolls.

1

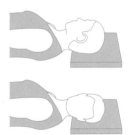

2. Test for: Shoulder rotation

Reach over your shoulder and attempt to reach to the top corner of your opposite shoulder blade (external rotation). Then reach behind your back and attempt to touch the lower part of the opposite shoulder blade (internal rotation).

Ideal range: External rotation: be able to reach and touch the top inside corner of the opposite shoulder.

Internal rotation: be able to reach behind and touch the lower angle of the opposite shoulder. Greater distance indicate the tighter the muscle.

Influence on your golf game: Tight external rotation on the right shoulder can lead to restriction of follow through. On the left shoulder will indicate tightness on the backswing.

Tightness on the left external rotators will have an impact on the flight of the ball.

2

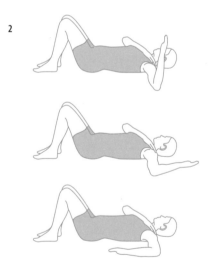

Pilates exercises: Floating arms, Four point challenge, diamond press, arm opening, arm circles, mid-back stretch, shoulder external rotation, shoulder internal rotation, shoulder push away, shoulder rowing, leg pull prone, Pilates push up.

3 Test for: Hamstring

Ideal range: Straighten your leg to a minimal distance of 70 degrees.

Influence on your golf game: Tightness leads to excessive flexion in the lumbar spine. Altered swing is also associated with overuse of the arms due to limitation in the trunk rotation/flexion.

Pilates exercises: Scissors, double leg stretch, leg circles, open leg rocker.

3

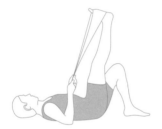

4 Test for: Waiter bow (lean forward standing)

This determines the length of the upper hamstrings and ability to achieve normal motion in the hips. Place both hands behind your back with the back of the hands flat against your back and fingers just touching. Bend forward with your knees locked.

Ideal range: Normal range is greater than 50 degrees before your fingers stop touching. Poor hamstring length means

4

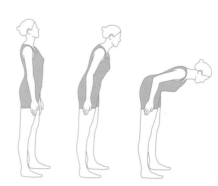

you will not be able to bend forward and maintain the lumbar curve in your spine.

Influence on your golf game: Swing faults (see chart on correct golf swing).

Pilates exercises: Hamstring lengthening, spinal curl, double leg stretch, lean forward bending.

5 Test for: Side bend

Stand with your feet hip-width apart, parallel against a wall. Slide your hand down your leg as far as you can go without your feet lifting off the ground.

5

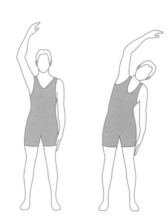

Ideal range: To reach the outside joint line of your knee.

Influence on your golf game: Swing faults (see chart on correct golf swing).

Pilates exercise: Side reach.

6 Test for: Thoracic extension lean forward standing

Stand with your back to a wall, about a foot distance away. Rest your buttocks, back, and head against the wall, keeping your knees soft. Allow your arms to float forward and up, while keeping your back in contact with the wall. Your back should not flatten as you raise your arms.

Ideal range: Arms should be able to touch the wall above your head without any trunk movement.

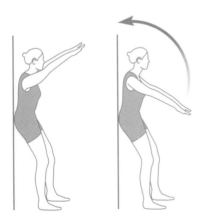

Influence on your golf game: Indicates if there is sufficient extension in the thoracic spine to protect your shoulders from injury during the golf swing.

Pilates exercises: Arm raises, swimming legs, spinal curls (arms only).

7 Test for: Spinal rotation

Lie on your back, knees bent and feet together. Rotate your legs to the side.

Ideal range: Your legs will lie flat on the floor without the opposite shoulder coming off the ground.

Influence on your golf game: Restricted spinal rotation will result in excessive shift and rotation of the hips during the back-swing and follow through. The shoulders will be overused to compensate.

Pilates exercises: Hip rolls, single knee kicks, arm opening, threading the needle, waist twists in standing.

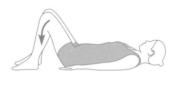

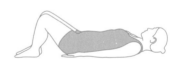

Pilates exercises to improve performance and prevent further injury

I Lengthen
▼ Balance
● Strengthen

CORE EXERCISES	Lower back pain	Golfer's shoulder	Golfer's elbow
curl up	●		●
diamond press	●	●	●
floating arms		●	
four point challenge	▼	▼	▼
hip opening	●		
static standing balance	▼		
FOUNDATION EXERCISES			
arm circles		●	●
arm opening		I ●	I ●
dart		I	●
hamstring lengthening	I		
long sitting stretch	●		
mid-back stretch		●	●
shoulder external rotation		●	●
shoulder internal rotation			●
shoulder push away			●
shoulder rowing		●	●
shoulder rotation control	●	I	●
side reach	●		
single knee kicks	I ●		

	Lower back pain	Golfer's shoulder	Golfer's elbow
spinal curls	●	●	●
T-band balance	▼		
threading the needle	●		I
PERFORMANCE PILATES			
bridging	●		
double leg stretch	●	I	
hundred		●	
leg pull prone	●	●	
lunge		●	
oblique curl up	●		
open leg rocker	●		
Pilates push up	●	●	
praying mantis		●	
rolling like ball	●		
scissors	I ●		
side kick series			
single leg stretch	●		
superman	●	●	
swimming	I ●	●	
waist twists in standing	●	●	I
wrist strengthening			●

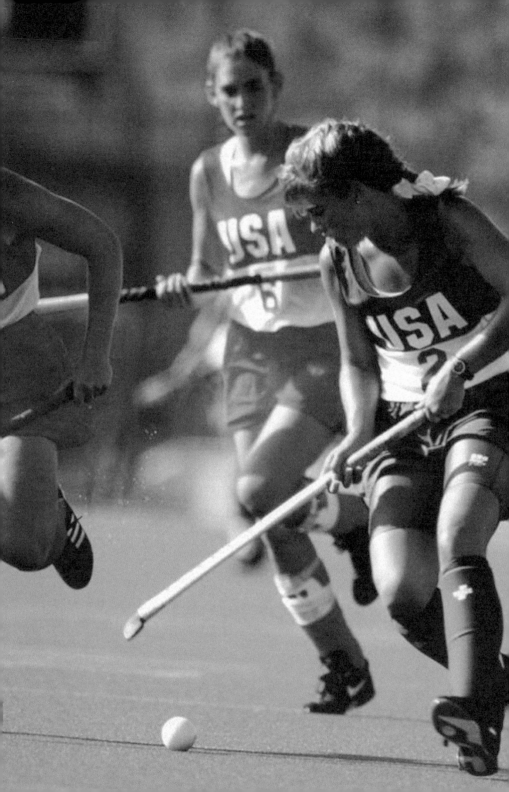

Hockey: Ice and Field

Ice hockey, one of the most popular team sports, is a fast-paced game in which a lot of players skate at high speed in a confined area. Players risk injury from high-impact collisions, both with each other and with the rigid boards that surround the rink. Field hockey can also be a high-impact game, resulting in mild to serious injuries. Most field hockey injuries, often sustained in the head area, are caused by a player being struck by a ball or stick. Both ice and field hockey require players to accelerate quickly in response to the puck or ball, and to change direction suddenly. These are the main causes of injuries to the ankle and knee.

Common hockey injuries

Low-back pain

Low-back pain tends to occur as a result of the playing position adopted during a hockey game. The pain tends to be non-specific in nature and centers on the lower back muscles.

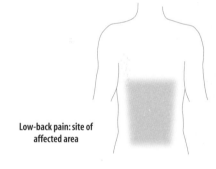

Low-back pain: site of affected area

Causes

A prolonged stooped position when dribbling and passing the ball.

Signs and symptoms

Generalized, dull aching pain in the lower back area, which tends to be aggravated by bending forward.

Pain may recede when the back is arched or stretched. Pain may not occur when resting.

Treatment

IMMEDIATE

If you have muscle spasms, apply ice for ten minutes or until the area is numbed.

Keep moving to help settle the pain.

If the pain persists for longer than three

days, it may be necessary to visit a chartered physiotherapist or osteopath.

LONG-TERM

Follow the recommended Pilates program at the end of this chapter.

How to prevent

Maintain length in the hip flexors (see page 99 to find out how to check the muscle length).

Achieve good core stability (see page 160 for the core stability program).

Ensure that you are fit to play your hockey game. Do not use the game to get you fit.

Ankle inversion injury

Ankle sprains are by far the most common injuries in sports. They're usually caused

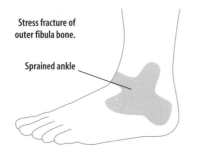

Stress fracture of outer fibula bone.

Sprained ankle

Ankle inversion injury: site of pain

by the ankle rolling over, forcing the foot into dorsiflexion and inversion.

Causes

Landing awkwardly from a jump.

Stepping or landing on your opponent's foot during the game.

Changing direction suddenly or a sudden deceleration during a run.

Running on an uneven surface.

Weak peroneal (ankle) muscles.

Tight Achilles tendon.

Existing ankle injury.

Signs and symptoms

You are able to describe the actual mechanism of injury.

The ankle hurts to touch, even at rest.

You are unable to walk without pain.

There is swelling and bruising on the side of the foot.

What sort of sprain do you have?

MILD SPRAIN

You do not limp when walking.

MODERATE SPRAIN

There is a noticeable limp when walking.

You cannot raise up on your toes or hop on your injured ankle.

SEVERE SPRAIN

Painful when placing weight on the injured foot.

You find it difficult to walk without any assistance.

Treatment

IMMEDIATE

P.R.I.C.E.

Bear weight on the ankle only when it is bearable.

Write the alphabet in the air with your foot to test range of pain-free motion.

LONG-TERM

Achieve a good sense of balance with the ankle (joint proprioception).

Build strength around the ankle joint.

Be sensitive to pain when you feel it.

Respect the pain during sport.

How to prevent

Maintain good strength and coordination around the ankle joint.

Follow the exercise program at the end of this chapter to improve your performance and prevent further ankle injuries.

Undergo fitness testing before commencing a hockey game to ensure your fitness levels are acceptable.

Warm up correctly before playing a hockey game.

Cool down, including stretching your entire body after playing.

Pay particular attention to stretching and warming up your ankles, hips, and lower back.

Acromioclavicular joint sprain

The acromioclavicular joint (AC) is vulnerable to injury in collision sports and in activities requiring repetitive overhead motions, such as upper-extremity strength training. The key to successful treatment is prompt and accurate recognition of the severity of AC injuries.

Causes

Falling onto your outstretched arm.

Repetitive overarm pitching.

Signs and symptoms

Pain, tendrness, or possible deformity around the AC.

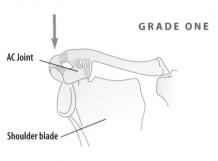

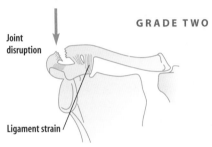

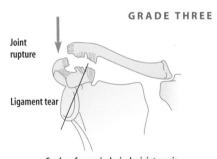

Grades of acromioclavicular joint sprain

Classification of pain

GRADE ONE PAIN

Symptoms: Pain or tenderness.

Treatment: Treat symptoms through P.R.I.C.E. Continue activity.

GRADE TWO PAIN

Symptoms: Pain, tenderness, and slight separation from the prominent end of the clavicle.

Treatment: Use a sling and rest for two to four weeks depending on severity.

GRADE THREE PAIN

Symptoms: Pain, tenderness, and marked separation of the joint from the prominent end of the clavicle.

Treatment: You may need to wear a brace and rest for six to eight weeks. Surgery may be necessary.

Knee injuries

During a hockey game the knee is put under large amounts of strain. It is reported to be the most serious site of injury. The injuries are caused by collisions, sudden twisting and direct impacts on the side of the knee.

Knee injuries can occur when the two collateral ligaments (medial and lateral ligaments) are damaged. The medial ligament is on the inside of the knee. The lateral ligament is on the outside of the knee and is meant to prevent the joint from gaping.

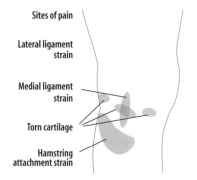

Sites of pain

Lateral ligament strain

Medial ligament strain

Torn cartilage

Hamstring attachment strain

For common knee injuries see medial ligament injury, anterior cruciate ligament injury, and meniscus tear, on pages 123–7.

Ulnar ligament tear

The ulnar collateral ligament helps to stablize the thumb joint as the thumb is pushed against the index and middle fingers, while gripping. Damage to it is fairly common in ice hockey.

Cause

Thumb is jammed back.

Signs and symptoms

Swelling and tenderness around thumb joint. Loss of grip using the thumb.

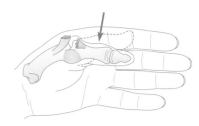

Ulnar ligament tear

Treatment

INITIAL

Comprehensive diagnosis of a tear.
Wear a thumb spica support or cast.

LONG-TERM

Avoid conflict during play.

How to prevent

Injury is avoidable by not engaging in fights on the ice or pulling an opponent's jersey during play.

Pilates exercises to improve performance and prevent further injury

▌ Lengthen
▼ Balance
● Strengthen

	Low back pain	Ankle inversion injury	Acromioclavicular joint sprain	Medial ligament	Anterior cruciate ligament	Meniscus tear	Ulnar ligament tear
CORE EXERCISES							
curl up	●			●	●	●	
diamond press			●				●
hip opening	●	●		●	●	●	
pelvic stability	●	●		●	●	●	
static standing balance	▼	▼		●▼	▼	▼	
FOUNDATION EXERCISES							
hamstring lengthening		●		▌	▌	▌	
long sitting stretch	●	●		●	●	●	
roll downs		▌●			●		
shoulder rotation							●
side reach	●				●		
single knee kicks	▌	▌●		▌	▌●	▌	
spinal curls	▌	●	●	●	●		
standing squat		●		●	●	●	
T-band balance	▼	▼		▼	▼	▼	
wall slides		▌●				●	
PERFORMANCE PILATES							
bridging		●		●	●	●	
lean forward bending		●					
lunge	●	●	●				
mermaid	●						
oblique curl up	●						
open leg rocker	●			▌●	●	●	
praying mantis	●		●		●		
rolling like a ball	●					●	
scissors	▌			●	●	●	
side kick series	●	●					
single leg stretch	●	●			●		
superman	●		●				
swimming	●		●	▌●	▌●	●	
tennis ball raises		●		●	●	●	
torpedo	●			●	●		
wrist strengthening							●

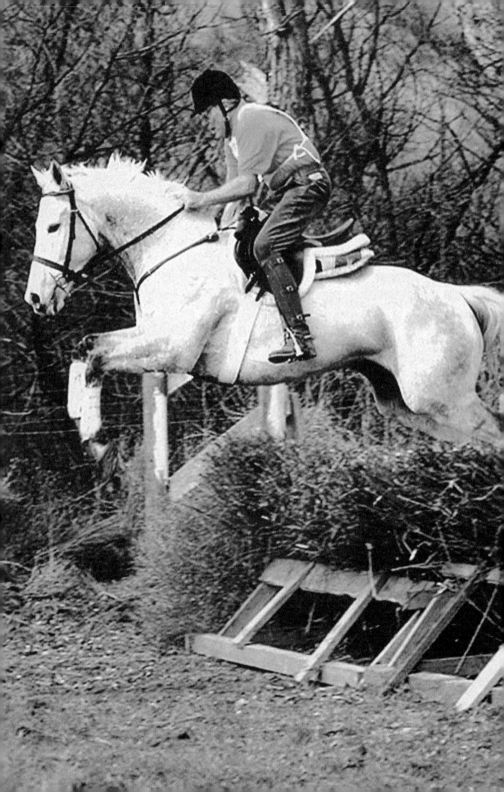

Horse Riding

Horse riding is a great form of exercise as it promotes good posture, tones the legs and strengthens the abdominals. Most injuries associated with horse riding arise from falling off a horse or during stable duties, such as mucking out. Around eighty percent of horse-related injuries occur while riding. These injuries respond particularly well to Pilates, as the practice improves basic skills, such as balance and postural awareness. These help to reduce the risk of falling. Pilates can also help increase your spatial awareness, which means you'll be able to act quickly when faced with the unpredictability of your horse.

INJURIES
—
SHOULDER PAIN
—
BACK PAIN
—
GROIN STRAIN
—

Common horse-riding injuries

Shoulder pain

Experiencing pain in the shoulder area while horse riding indicates the presence of postural problems, usually because you are slumping your shoulders and failing to tighten your abdominal muscles while riding.

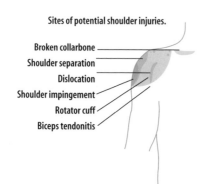

Sites of potential shoulder injuries.

Broken collarbone
Shoulder separation
Dislocation
Shoulder impingement
Rotator cuff
Biceps tendonitis

Causes

Bowing the head while riding. Hold your head high at all times to prevent the cervical spine becoming stiff.

Holding arms and elbows at an awkward position. The rider's arms should loosely hang close to the sides.

Poor control of the horse may strain the shoulder area.

Signs and symptoms

Pain in the upper shoulder area.

Pain in the mid-back area.

Treatment

IMMEDIATE

Reduce the tension in the neck and shoulder areas (upper trapezius muscles) by applying a hot water bottle to the neck for 15 minutes.

Maintain range of motion and flexibility in the neck. See neck rolls (page 187).

Raise your postural awareness.

Be aware of stretching and rotating your neck while riding, so that it doesn't become stiff in one position.

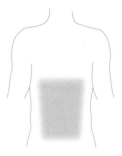

If you attempt to lift your leg to 90 degrees while experiencing back pain you will feel a restriction in the hip and lower back area and the pain will usually limit your movement to a range of only 60 degrees.

Back pain

Back pain is quite common in horse riders as a result of incorrect posture and the continuous motion of the activity which can jar or injure a weak or incorrectly aligned back.

How to handle a horse

Before you mount the horse

Let your horse know where you are at all times. Exercise caution when at the rear of the horse.

Do not hold reins or ropes in a loop on or around your hand, as they may trap and injure your fingers.

While riding

Choose your mount carefully. Make sure it is suited to your capabilities.

Never ride bareback unless you are competent to do so.

Learn to control the horse before leaving the safety of the paddock.

Travel in single file along the road.

Always leave at least one horse's distance between your own and other mounts.

If riding through water, kick your feet out of the stirrups in case you fall.

Causes

If the rider is unable to adopt various positions or postures during the activity, and adapt to a wide variety of conditions (walking, cantering, and galloping) he or she may strain or jar his/her back. The rider should sit as far forward on the saddle as he or she comfortably can. Sitting incorrectly will place more strain on the lower back muscles.

Finding your center of gravity while sitting on the horse allows you to shift your weight to the appropriate side when changing direction. You can find your center of gravity on the horse by placing your pelvis in a neutral position, then tilting it forward when moving. This posture will alleviate any strain on the muscles and soft tissue in the pelvic area.

Finding neutral pelvis position

The deep abdominal muscles need to coordinate with the superficial muscles in order to achieve a correct pelvis tilt. The back muscles (latissimus dorsi) also need to remain strong and controlled to aid the abdominals and upper arms (see page 160).

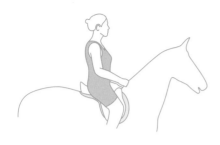

Correct seating position.

Groin strain

Groin strain is a common problem among many people who ride horses. It affects the hip adductors and commonly occurs when there is forced side-to-side motion.

High forces occur in the adductor tendons when the rider must shift to the opposite direction suddenly. As a result, the adductor muscles contract to generate opposing forces.

Signs and symptoms

A deep, dull ache which intensifies with the tilt of the pelvis.

Treatment

IMMEDIATE

Establish strength and control in the deep abdominal muscles (transversus abdominis).

Establish the correct length and strength of your back muscles (latissimus dorsi).

Have your sitting balance properly assessed while riding.

LONG-TERM

Maintain length in the back (latissimus dorsi) by including the following exercises in your Pilates routine:

Diamond press (page 170). Side reach (page 194). Double leg stretch (page 205).

How to prevent

Establish good control of the core areas—trunk, pelvis, and shoulders. This will help you to easily maintain a good sitting posture without causing tension in the shoulders.

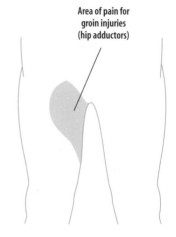

Area of pain for groin injuries (hip adductors)

Groin injuries: site of pain.

Causes

Constantly shifting your weight in the saddle in order to achieve a comfortable sitting position can place strain on the adductor muscles. Long periods of horse riding may also cause strain as the muscle has been sustained in a lengthened position for an extended amount of time.

Signs and symptoms

Dull ache to the adductor muscle (groin and inner thigh) develops over 24 to 48 hours after horse riding.

Treatment

IMMEDIATE

Reduce the extent of the muscle soreness by warming down after riding.

Massage the area to help relax the muscles and prevent stiffness.

Follow the Pilates program outlined at the end of this chapter.

Anti-inflammatories may help to relieve muscle pain.

Some Pilates movements will help to keep the muscles flexible. See pelvic stability (page 175).

LONG-TERM

Regular massage to the adductor muscles will help prevent tenderness.

To maintain strength in the hip adductors (muscles that allow the hips to move from side to side) include roll downs (page 188) in your Pilates program.

How to prevent

Ensure that your muscles have the required lengthening and strengthening abilities required to undertake this activity. See the abdominal training test (page 161) to check your abdominal strength. Strong abdominals will help you to maintain a strong core and prevent your posture from slumping while horse riding.

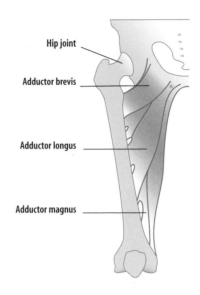

Hip joint

Adductor brevis

Adductor longus

Adductor magnus

Groin injuries: affected areas.

Pilates exercises to improve performance and prevent further injury

▌ Lengthen
▼ Balance
● Strengthen

CORE EXERCISES	Shoulder pain	Back pain	Groin strain
curl up	●	●	
diamond press	●	▌	
floating arms	●	●	
four point challenge	▼	▼	▼
hip opening		●	●
imprinting	●	●	
pelvic stability			●
neutral spine	●	●	●
static standing balance			▼

FOUNDATION EXERCISES	Shoulder pain	Back pain	Groin strain
arm opening	●		
big squeeze		●	▌
dart	●		
hamstring lengthening			▌
mid-back stretch	▌●		
neck rolls	▌●		
roll downs			●
shoulder internal rotation	●		
shoulder external rotation	●		
shoulder push away	●		
shoulder rowing	●		
side reach	●	▌	●
single knee kick			▌
spinal curls			●
star			●
T-band balance			▼
threading the needle	●		●
wall slides			●
windows	●		

PERFORMANCE PILATES	Shoulder pain	Back pain	Groin strain
bridging		●	●
double leg stretch	●	●	
hundred		●	
lean forward bending	●		
leg pullback			●
mermaid	●		
oblique curl up			●
open leg rocker			▼●
praying mantis	●		
rolling like a ball	●		
scissors		●	●
side kick series			●
side rolls			●
single leg stretch			●
sitting knee folds		●	
superman	●	●	
swimming			●
torpedo			●

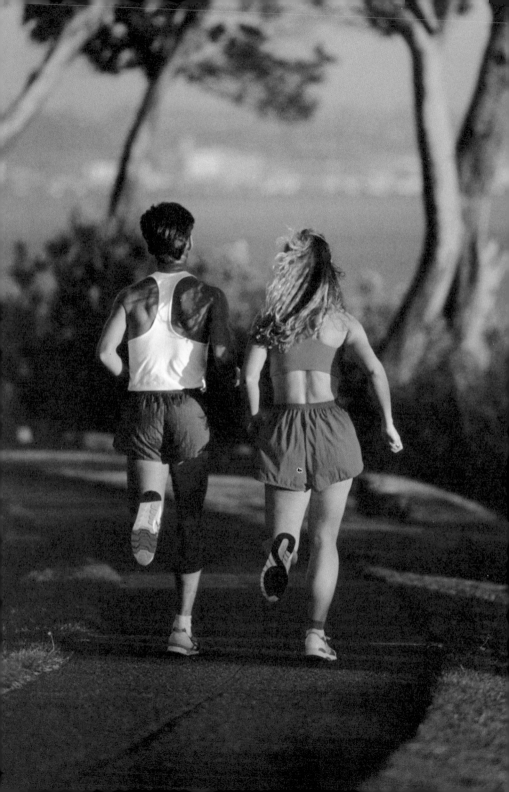

Running

Running is a great aerobic exercise that gives the heart and lungs a good workout. It also involves the entire body, strengthening the legs and firming the buttocks, stomach, and upper body. It is an exercise that almost anyone can do, anywhere, at any time: all you need is some open space and a pair of running shoes. It is an ideal weight-bearing exercise as it helps to increase bone density in the skeleton, which is necessary to avoid osteoporosis and thinning of the bones in later life. The most common injuries occur in the lower limbs (calves, ankles, Achilles tendon) and lower back. These problems occur due to poor technique, uneven surfaces, muscle overuse, excessive training, or incorrect footwear. Running along on hard surfaces can, in time, cause muscle strain and damage to the joints. Pilates for runners aims specifically to help strengthen the lower back, reducing pressure caused by the constant jarring on the spine during a run.

INJURIES

SCIATICA

PIRIFORMIS SYNDROME

ILIOTIBIAL BAND SYNDROME

HAMSTRING STRAIN

PATELLOFEMORAL PAIN

CALF MUSCLE STRAIN

SHIN SPLINTS

STRESS FRACTURE

ACHILLES TENDONITIS

ANKLE INVERSION INJURY

PLANTAR FASCIITIS

Common running injuries

Sciatica

Sciatica is the term given to pain down the leg, which is caused by irritation of the main nerve into the leg, the sciatic nerve. This pain tends to be caused where the nerves pass through and emerge from the lower bones of the spine (lumbar vertebrae). The exact cause of sciatica is not fully understood, but can involve a slipped or herniated disk. This means one of the disks, that lie between each of the vertebrae in the lower back (lumbar area), has cracked and allowed some of the inner disk material to

protrude, putting pressure on the adjacent nerve root, the sciatic nerve. Sciatica tends to be accompanied by back pain.

Causes

Poor posture is one of the main causes of sciatica. If one leg is longer than the other, you may be overcompensating the shorter leg by leaning too heavily to one side. This can place pressure on the lower back and ultimately the sciatic nerve.

Signs and symptoms

Pain will be felt below the knee and it may be difficult to run as normal.

Pain is felt as a constant, intense ache that does not improve with bed rest.

There may be limited flexibility of the lumbar region when bending forward or to the side.

Seek medical attention if you experience any of the following:

Inability to fall asleep, or waking early in the morning.

Fever or unexplained high temperature.

Cauda equina syndrome, which causes bowel or bladder problems.

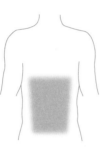

If you attempt to lift your leg to 90 degrees whilst experiencing back pain you will feel a restriction in the hip and lower back area and the pain will usually limit your movement to a range of only 60 degrees.

Bilateral lower limb pain or saddle paranaesthesia, which is an "altered" feeling in the area of your groin.

Treatment

IMMEDIATE

Anti-inflammatories can help to relieve constant pain.

Exercising little and often. Prolonged periods of bedrest will only worsen the symptoms.

Seek advice from a chartered physiotherapist or osteopath.

LONG-TERM

Follow a Pilates program to reestablish muscle support for the spine.

Always warm up your entire body with stretches before running.

Pay attention to your posture when you run. Keep your core muscles strong and tight (see page 160).

Piriformis syndrome

Piriformis syndrome is a condition in which the piriformis muscle irritates the sciatic nerve and causes pain in the buttocks and sometimes along the back of the leg and into the foot. The sciatic nerve passes through the sciatic notch below the piriformis muscle.

If the muscle gets tight then the nerve is compressed and it will become inflamed

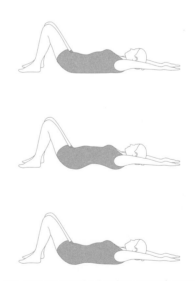

Lying in the psoas position (knee bent up to 90 degrees at the hip and knees, in a supported position), engage the spine in the neutral position in order to engage the muscles that support the back.

and cause pain. This condition is most common among women, and is thought to be common among active individuals (such as runners and hikers).

A common cause of piriformis syndrome is having tight adductor muscles (inside your thigh). This means the abductors on the outside cannot work properly and so put more strain on the piriformis.

Causes

Minor twisting on one leg may be caused by incorrect running style or relying too heavily on one leg.

A difference in leg length can also cause muscular pain. To find out whether your legs are of slightly different lengths, measure from two points—the anterior superior iliac spine (front bony point of the pelvis) and the belly button, to the inside of the ankle. Compare the results to see if there is a possible difference in your leg length. However, this may not necessarily be the cause of your problem.

A weak piriformis muscle. Stand on one leg with your hip slightly rotated outward. The muscle is weak if the leg turns inward at the hip.

Signs and symptoms

Pain felt in the buttock in the adjacent piriformis muscle.

Pain or numbness down the leg.

Pain when the muscle is contracted and irritation when the hip is externally rotated.

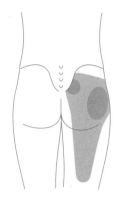
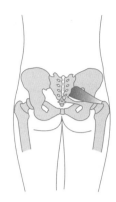
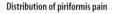

Distribution of piriformis pain   Location of piriformis muscle

Treatment

IMMEDIATE

Pain-relieving medication.

Avoid running until your symptoms are under control.

LONG-TERM

The following exercises can help to strengthen the piriformis muscle:

1. Try running in the swimming pool wearing an aqua vest.

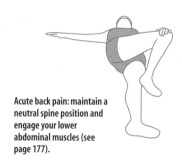

Acute back pain: maintain a neutral spine position and engage your lower abdominal muscles (see page 177).

2. Strengthen the gluteus medius muscle. See hip opening exercise (page 174).

3. Lengthen the psoas muscle by doing single knee kicks (see page 195).

4. Stretching the piriformis internally by rotating and adducting a flexed hip.

5. Do knee drops. This will stretch your external hip rotators, gluteus maximus, obturator internus, gluteus medius/minimus, psoas, obturator externus, and piriformis.

6. When you return to your running program, stick to even surfaces.

How to prevent

Try to avoid turning your hips inward when you are running, particularly when training on slopes.

Correct leg length discrepancy. Visit a qualified physiotherapist or podiatrist for a professional assessment.

Iliotibial band syndrome

Iliotibial band syndrome is one of the leading causes of lateral knee pain in runners. The iliotibial band is a superficial thickening of tissue on the outside of the thigh, extending from the outside of the pelvis, over the hip and knee, and inserting just below the knee. The band is crucial to stabilizing the knee during running, moving from behind the femur to the front of it during a running stride.

Causes

Running too much too soon, without sufficient fitness.

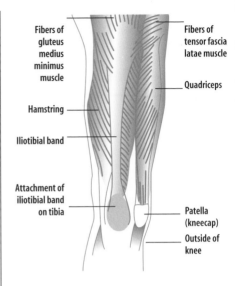

Fibers of gluteus medius minimus muscle

Fibers of tensor fascia latae muscle

Quadriceps

Hamstring

Iliotibial band

Attachment of iliotibial band on tibia

Patella (kneecap)

Outside of knee

Iliotibial band syndrome has the same symptoms as tronchanteric gluteal pain, but the pain is caused by the inflammation of the actual iliotibial band because it is tight. There is also friction of the band on the greater trochanter (the outside of the hip joint).

A tight iliotibial tract which is brought on by "bowing" knees and/or foot pronation or flat feet (feet turning inwards). This can lead to the lower limb turning inward.

A fall onto the hip.

Signs and symptoms

Pain is localized to the greater trochanter on the lateral aspect of the hip (often experienced by long-distance runners).

The inflammation is aggravated by hip movements (for example, when running or getting out of the car).

There is a catching or snapping of the bursa (the fluid-filled sac in this area) across the greater trochanter.

There is pain and tenderness over the trochanter. Pain increases with any weight-bearing movements.

Other diagnosis

If you are concerned about pain in this area see a medical professional to make an accurate diagnosis. This injury can sometimes be a stress fracture of the neck femur or referred pain from the spine and/or the sacroiliac joint.

You can test for a strain in the iliotibial band by trying Ober's test (see page 45).

Treatment

IMMEDIATE

Stretch out the iliotibial band.

Run shorter distances.

Avoid running up or down hills.

Take anti-inflammatory tablets to reduce the pain.

Tape the gluteal area if the problem is very painful and causing you irritation.

Regularly do the stretching and strengthening exercises recommended at the end of this chapter to minimize your symptoms.

LONG-TERM

When you return to regular running, avoid going along steep cambers on the road. Keep to flat surfaces and build up your distance on the flat.

Alter your training schedule if the pain is present only during running.

Try reducing your running distance by half if you are still experiencing problems.

The following exercises can help to strengthen the iliotibial band:

1. Stretch abductors of the hip—the gluteus medius and tensor fasciae latae muscles (see page 163).

2. Stretch gluteus maximus, gluteus minimus, piriformis, and obturator internus muscles (see page 163).

3. Strengthen the muscles around the hip (see page 163).

How to prevent

Maintain the ratio between the length and strength of the muscles around the hip, particularly the gluteus medius and deep hip rotators by undertaking the Pilates program detailed at the end of this chapter.

Gradually build up your training program. Don't overdo it too soon.

Hamstring strain

This is the most common injury suffered by runners and athletes in general.

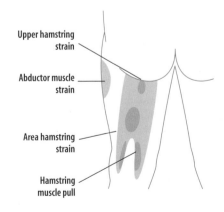

Upper hamstring strain

Abductor muscle strain

Area hamstring strain

Hamstring muscle pull

Sites of pain.

The hamstring is actually a group of three muscles that help to straighten (extend) the leg at the hip and bend (flex) the leg at the knee. The pull felt during an injury is a strain or tear in the muscles or tendons.

Causes

ACUTE STRAIN

For runners, acute hamstring strain can occur when the runner increases the intensity of springing.

Contributing factors are:

Cold weather. Make sure you warm up your muscles to avoid strain.

Fatigue. Don't push your body when it is feeling the strain of training.

Muscle weakness can occur when placed under tension. This usually happens when endurance runners sprint or slip.

Running when you have an existing injury.

Tight neurological tissue as a result of restricted movement in the lumbar spine. If you do suffer from tightness in this area, you will need a detailed assessment from a medical practitioner.

CHRONIC STRAIN

Inadequate hamstring length indicated by tightness of the muscle.

Inadequate strength and flexibility in the hip rotator.

Increasing mileage too dramatically or changing running style.

Signs and symptoms

ACUTE

Increased inflexibility of the hamstrings.

Localized tenderness in the muscle.

Bruising at the back of the knee owing to muscle fibers tearing and bleeding.

Pain on bending to touch the toes.

CHRONIC

Soreness where the tissue has not completely healed, which indicates loss of elasticity within the muscle.

Treatment

IMMEDIATE

Place an ice pack on the affected muscle for ten minutes or until the area is numb.

Gently contract and relax the muscle.

Tape the muscle to prevent any overpull on the fibers.

Take anti-inflammatory tablets to reduce pain and swelling.

LONG-TERM

Start jogging slowly to test for any pain.

The Pilates program at the end of this chapter aims to coordinate the muscles.

Patellofemoral pain (also called Runner's knee)

Runner's knee occurs as a result of softening and changes to the undersurface of the kneecap. It is caused by a functional imbalance of the quadriceps muscles which controls the movement of the patella in the femoral groove.

Causes

Overtraining, bending, squatting, and kneeling can lead to the vastus medialis muscle wasting away meaning that the

Patellofemoral pain

Chondomalacia patellae

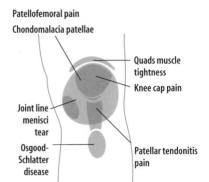

Quads muscle tightness

Knee cap pain

Joint line menisci tear

Osgood-Schlatter disease

Patellar tendonitis pain

patellar bone drifts outward and causes friction against the outside of the femur bone (lateral femoral condyle).

Biomechanical malalignment in the knee.

Genu valgum (knock knees)

Genu varum (bow legs).

Tibia valga, turning of the lower shin outward when running.

Mid-foot over pronation/flat feet. Occurs when the medial arch of the foot is flattened and weight is placed on the entire surface of the foot, which in turn places extra stress on the knee joint and tibia.

Valgus heel. This is rare but may occur following a severe inversion injury of the ankle (see page 96).

Wasting of the quadriceps muscle.

Tension in the iliotibial band as a result of an imbalance along the band from the muscles at the top—the gluteus medius and minimus.

Hyper-extending the knee (locking the knee backward).

Signs and symptoms

Anterior knee pain as a result of exercise.

Pain or soreness after sitting with bent knees for some time.

Excessive bending in the knees.

Pain may grip the knee after running for a few miles. It may recede with rest, then recur when you start running again.

Pain in the patellofemoral crepitus (the joint formed by the kneecap on the knee bone).

Pain while contracting the quadriceps.

Pain during weight-bearing sports.

Pain as a result of repeated knee flexion/extension.

The pain is vague and nonspecific.

Tenderness in the medial side of the patella (inside aspect of the knee cap).

Small amount of swelling in the knee.

Muscles giving way due to quadriceps inhibition (a reflex that releases the hold on the muscle due to pain).

Patellofemoral joint—movement may be restricted or you may feel a "giving way" sensation in the knee cap).

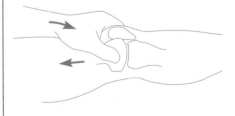

Clarke's test
Hold the kneecap still while contracting the quadriceps. If you feel pain, the test is positive.

Muscles involved

Gastrocnemius
Hamstrings
Rectus femoris
Iliotibial band
Soft tissue
Lateral retinaculum
Iliotibial band
Vastus lateralis
Vastus medialis obliques
Hip abductors/external
rotators (gluteus medius)

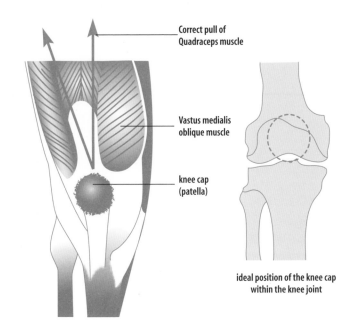

Correct pull of
Quadraceps muscle

Vastus medialis
oblique muscle

knee cap
(patella)

ideal position of the knee cap
within the knee joint

Squatting can be painful in the front aspect of the knee joint.

Treatment

IMMEDIATE

P.R.I.C.E.

Complete the wall sides exercises (page 201) and knee bends (page 175).

Apply tape to improve the tracking and support of the knee.

LONG-TERM

Hip stabilizing. See exercise plan at the end of this chapter.

Quadriceps strengthening (see page 214).

PREVENTION

Maintain strength in the quadriceps muscle, particularly the vastus medialis oblique (the muscle inside your knee). Keep a good sense of balance in the muscle, by working on your single leg balance exercises (see page 225).

Maintain muscle control through the pelvis and pelvic stability (see page 175).

Calf muscle strain

The calf muscles consist of the gastrocnemius, which is the big muscle at the back of the lower leg and the soleus muscle, which is a smaller muscle lower down in the leg and under the gastrocnemius. Either of these two muscles can be strained or torn. A sudden sharp pain in the calf muscle followed by difficulty using it usually indicates calf strain. The most common place to get this injury is roughly halfway between the knee and the heel. You can test for this by contracting the muscle against resistance with the legs straight. Pain is felt midway up the calf muscle.

Causes

Failing to warm up properly before a run.

Repetitive slapping down of foot while the knee is extended. Pain is usually immediately felt in the calf muscle.

Excessive lunging when not warmed up.

Suddenly ceasing activity, such as stopping running, without warming down correctly.

Signs and symptoms

Sudden sharp pain in the calf muscle.

Being unable to continue with activity.

Treatment

IMMEDIATE

Undertake the P.R.I.C.E. recovery plan. Apply ice for ten minutes immediately after feeling the pain.

Reduce the amount of weight on the leg by using a crutch or resting.

Use a heel raise in your shoe if you are unable to walk on a flat surface without experiencing sharp pain.

Maintain a range of motion exercises— but do not perform any movements that stretch the calf muscle.

Flex the foot backward and forward (active dorsiflexion/plantar flexion) to test for pain.

LONG-TERM

Resume exercising only when pain has completely diminished. Enter into moderate activity only when tolerable.

How to prevent

Warm up adequately for your run.

Follow the lengthening program for calf muscles at the end of this chapter.

Shin splints

Shin splints is the term commonly used to describe lower leg pain which is non-specific in nature. If you suffer from shin splints it is possible that you experience one or all of the following injuries:

1. Stress fracture to the shin bone as a result of overtraining and abnormal stress on the bone.
2. Compartment syndrome—an acute or sharp pain localized inside the border of the tibia or the muscle in the lower leg. It is caused by the muscle bulking up inside its containing tissue as a result of sporting activity (rather like putting too much in to a carrier bag so that it feels as though it may split).
3. Muscle imbalance. The presence of an imbalance between the muscles in the lower leg and the muscles that work around the foot (peroneal muscles, tibialis anterior/posterior).

Signs and symptoms

PAIN RELATED TO EXERCISE

Constantly increasing.

Worse on impact.

Decreases with warm up.

Increases with exercise.

Decreases with rest.

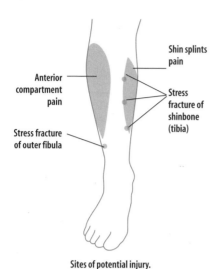

Shin splints pain

Anterior compartment pain

Stress fracture of shinbone (tibia)

Stress fracture of outer fibula

Sites of potential injury.

OTHER SYMPTOMS

Night ache increases in the morning.

Pain is worse after you have exercised.

Causes

Sudden increase in training.

Running on hard surfaces.

Muscle fatigue leading to stress upon your tibia.

Inadequate footwear.

Increasing exercise intensity too rapidly.

Poor biomechanics during running.

Repetitive jumping.

Prolonged exercise bouts.

Muscle/fascia compartment size.

Treatment

IMMEDIATE

Apple ice to the tender area as soon as you feel any pain. Move the ice around the tender area for ten minutes.

Rest for two to three weeks until the pain dissipates.

When you begin training again, run on a softer surface.

Make sure you're wearing the correct shoes for your foot and training needs.

If the muscle is inflamed, complete the stretching program at the end of this chapter.

How to prevent

Always get expert advice on the correct footwear for your training needs.

Warm up properly before commencing any exercise.

Concentrate on increasing your flexibility in your lower limbs.

Follow the Pilates program at the end of this chapter to strengthen your lower limbs.

Stress fracture

Stress fracture of the tibia begins with gradual onset of shin pain. The pain is aggravated when exercise compounds the failure in the structure of the bone.

Causes

A change in the ability to absorb impact during training.

Repetitive changes in the bone due to overloading on the bone, caused by excessive training.

Signs and symptoms

Pain may occur when walking, at rest, or even at night.

Tenderness, localized over the tibia bone.

A medical practitioner needs to assess the full extent of damage, usually by a bone scan.

Treatment

IMMEDIATE

Rest from all pain-creating activities.

Run in water with an aqua vest to maintain your fitness levels, but several weeks of rest may be necessary before you start running on hard surfaces again.

LONG-TERM

Once you do not experience any pain when walking, gradually start your training program, slowly building up the amount of exercise you do.

While the pain is present do cross-training—basically activities such as riding or swimming and any activities that are low-impact.

How to prevent

Keep a diary of your training to determine whether you are doing too much. These notes will help you pinpoint when and where the pain occurs during specific training sessions.

Achilles tendonitis

The Achilles tendon, the largest tendon in the body, connects the gastrocnemius and soleus muscles to the heel, transferring the force of their contractions to lift the heel. There are two types of Achilles tendonitis: one is an inflammatory condition that occurs because of overuse, the other involves degeneration of the tendons.

Causes

Turning the foot over while running.

Straining the Achilles tendon while jumping or landing suddenly.

Many years spent jumping or running.

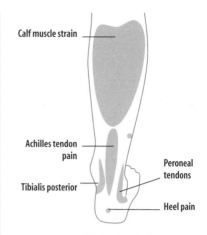

Ankle injuries: sites of pain.

Inadequate fitness.

Running on a different surface.

A change in footwear.

Calf weakness.

Tight gastrocnemius muscle.

Restriction when lifting foot upward.

Excessive pronation of the ankle and foot, causing the Achilles tendon to pull off-center and become inflamed.

Signs and symptoms

A severe, burning pain in the tendon area.

Pain and/or stiffness in the tendon first thing in the morning.

Tenderness makes the area uncomfortable to touch. There is also often a deep, marked swelling that moves with the tendon.

Treatment

IMMEDIATE

Stop running while the tendon is tender, or if you experience any pain as you raise up on your toes.

Take anti-inflammatory tablets to reduce pain and tenderness.

Gentle heel raises can help to resolve the acute condition in three to four weeks.

LONG-TERM

Follow the "Immediate" treatments until pain settles.

Undertake a muscle strengthening program to lengthen the ankle muscles under tension (see heel drop on page 207).

How to prevent

Stretch out the calf and hamstring muscles by pulling the foot upward.

Practice tensing your lower leg to lengthen the Achilles tendon (see heel drop on page 207).

Ankle inversion injury

Ankle sprains are by far the most common injuries in sports. They are usually caused by the ankle rolling over, forcing the foot into dorsiflexion and inversion.

Causes

Landing awkwardly from a jump.

Changing direction suddenly or sudden deceleration during running.

Running on an uneven surface.

Weak peronea (ankle) muscles.

Tight Achilles tendon.

Existing ankle injury.

Signs and symptoms

Being able to pinpoint the exact location and feeling of the injury.

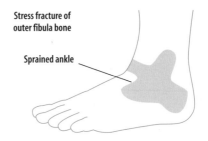

Stress fracture of outer fibula bone

Sprained ankle

Diagram of area affected.

Feeling a popping sensation.

Feeling a tearing sensation, followed by a sharp pain.

The ankle is painful to touch.

Swelling or bruising on side of the foot.

Being unable to walk without feeling some pain.

Treatment

IMMEDIATE

Control pain and swelling through the following procedure:

P.R.I.C.E.

Bear weight only when it is tolerable.

Write the alphabet in the air with your foot to test the range of pain-free motion.

LONG-TERM

Achieve a good sense of balance with the ankle (see proprioception page 13).

Build strength around the ankle joint.

Be sensitive to pain when you feel it.

How to prevent

Maintain good strength and coordination around the ankle joint.

Follow the exercise program on pages 98–99 to improve your performance and prevent further ankle injury.

Plantar fasciitis

Plantar fasciitis, which may cause the heel to hurt, feel hot, or swell, is an inflammation of the plantar fascia, a thin layer of tough tissue supporting the arch of the foot. Repeated microscopic tears of the plantar fascia cause pain. Sometimes plantar fasciitis is associated with "heel spurs"; this is not always accurate, as bony growths on the heel may or may not be a factor.

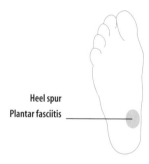

Heel spur
Plantar fasciitis

Site of pain.

Causes

Overstretching of plantar fascia because of poor foot posture, prolonged standing, or excessive running.

Wearing shoes with inadequate arch support (see correct footwear page 16).

Flexible arches of the foot.

Tight Achilles tendon.

Signs and symptoms

One-sided pain on the sole of the foot.

Pain when getting out of bed.

Pain during initial weight-bearing in morning, which is aggravated with activity.

Treatment

IMMEDIATE

Apply ice to the tender area for ten minutes or until the area is numb.

Use a heel raise in your shoe.

LONG-TERM

Integrate foot muscle strengthening exercises into your training program.

Use a heel pad in your shoe.

Make sure you have the correct footwear.

How to prevent

Make sure that you have good flexibility in your lower limbs.

Your footwear should have a supportive arch and be suitable for the type of training you are doing.

Training tips

Make sure you are wearing the correct shoes for your feet. If your feet roll inward you require different shoes.

When warming up concentrate on stretching the hip flexors, hamstrings, ligaments, quadriceps, and the lower back.

Comprehensive warm-up benefits

Increases the body temperature in your muscles.

Increases blood flow and oxygen to the muscles.

Increases the speed of nerve impulses.

Increases range of motion of the joints, which reduces the risk of tearing muscles and ligaments.

Pilates exercises to improve performance and prevent further injury

I Lengthen
▼ Balance
● Strength

	Sciatica	Piriformis syndrome	Iliotibial band syndrome	Hamstring strain	Patellofemoral pain	Shin splints	Ankle inversion injury	Achilles tendonitis	Plantar fasciitis
CORE EXERCISES									
curl up	●	●	●	●				●	●
four point challenge	▼	▼	▼	▼	▼				
hip opening	●	●	I ●	●			●	●	I ●
imprinting	●								
pelvic stability	I ●	●	●	●	●	●	●	●	●
neutral spine	●								
static standing balance			I	▼	▼	▼		▼	▼
FOUNDATION EXERCISES									
big squeeze		●	●	●	●				
dart				●					
hamstring lengthening					I		●	I	
hamstring stretch	I								
long sitting stretch						●	●	●	
roll downs	●		●		●	I	●	I	I
side reach	●	●		●					
single knee kick	I	I	I ●	●	●	I	●		I
spinal curls	●	●	●	●		●	●	I ●	I
standing squat		●	●	●	●	●	●	●	●
T-band balance		▼	I	▼	▼	▼		▼	▼
wall slides		●		●	●	I ●	●	I ●	I ●

PERFORMANCE PILATES

	Sciatica	Piriformis syndrome	Iliotibial band syndrome	Hamstring strain	Patellofemoral pain	Shin splints	Ankle inversion injury	Achilles tendonitis	Plantar fasciitis
bridging	●	●	●	●	●		●	●	●
double leg stretch		●	●	●	●			●	
heel drop							●		
hundred	●	●	●	●	●			●	
lean forward bending					●			●	
lunge							●	●	
oblique curl ups	●								
open leg rocker			▌		●			●	
praying mantis		●	●	●					
roll up		●	●	●		●			
rolling like a ball	▌							▌	
scissors	▌				●			▌●	▌
shoulder challenge									
side kick series			●	●	●	●	●	●	
side rolls		●		●					
single leg stretch	▌●		●		●	●	●	▌●	
sitting knee folds		●	●	●				●	
swimming	●	●	●	●	●	●		●	▌
tennis ball raises					●	●	●	●	
torpedo		●	●	●				●	
wrist strengthening		●							

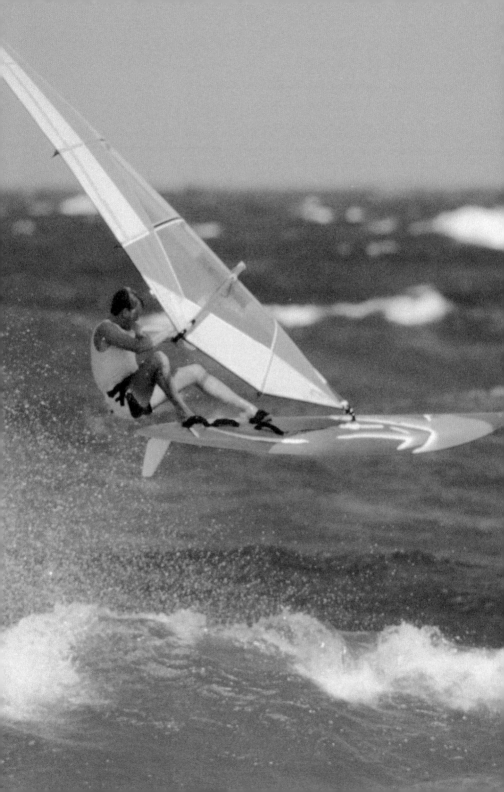

Sailing and Windsurfing

Sailing and windsurfing are strenuous sports that involve the entire body. You need to be extremely fit, with muscular strength, in order to endure the strenuous pressures of competition racing and handling heavy equipment. Such vigorous activity can lead to injuries, which specifically relate to the posture you adopt while sailing. For example, the "sewer" person—the person responsible for packing the sails—tends to be more susceptible to problems in the lumbar spine area because of the forward bending, and constant rotating of the spine required to drag and pack the sails. The "grinder," or winch man, is more susceptible to upper-body injuries as well as lower back problems. These are caused by the constant bending forward and the high-speed motions required to move the winch handles. Although windsurfing is a solo sport, injuries can occur as a result of falls, upper-body strain, and sudden changes in direction.

Common sailing and windsurfing injuries

Sailor's shoulder

Owing to the repetitive overhead movements used when sailing and windsurfing, the shoulder area tends to suffer from several painful injuries. These include rotator-cuff pain, tenderness in the tendons of the biceps, and impingement problems.

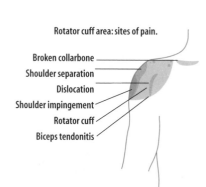

Rotator cuff area: sites of pain.

Broken collarbone

Shoulder separation

Dislocation

Shoulder impingement

Rotator cuff

Biceps tendonitis

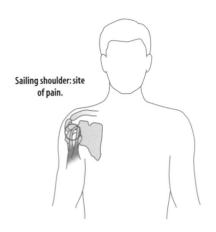

Sailing shoulder: site of pain.

Treatment

IMMEDIATE

Pinpoint the cause of the problem in order to avoid aggravating the condition.

Apply ice to the front of your shoulder joint for ten minutes, or until the area is numb.

Use anti-inflammatories as prescribed by your medical practitioner.

LONG-TERM

It is important to determine the underlying cause of injury, so that you know whether the problem is a result of imbalance, an impingement of the shoulder joint or instability. If you suspect the injury is instability, perform the apprehension test on page 134.

Correct your posture when bending and reaching.

Tape the affected area. This will help keep the shoulder stable and avoid further injury.

Follow a strengthening program specially designed for the upper body. See the Pilates strengthening program on page 108.

Shoulder dislocation

A shoulder dislocation is when the top part of the arm bone (humeral head) slips out of its socket (glenoid cavity). Forward (anterior) dislocations are most common. When this occurs the anterior inferior labrum (a piece of cartilage that stabilizes the shoulder) frequently is torn. Shoulder dislocations can also occur backward (posterior) and downward (inferior).

Causes

A dislocation can occur when the arm is forcibly moved into an awkward position during a fall or forced pulling on a joint. If a dislocation or partial dislocation (known as a subluxation) occurs with only minor force, the injury may be caused by multidirectional instability.

Signs and symptoms

Loss of active range of movement in the shoulder joint in most directions.

Feeling your joint "pop out."

If you experience pain in your shoulder when you move your arm out to the side this indicates a positive impingement test.

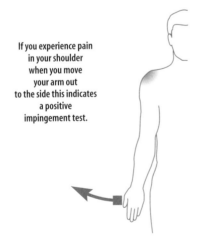

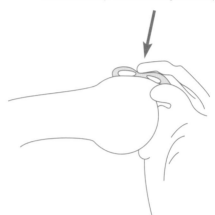

A shoulder dislocation is when the top part of the arm bone (humeral head) slips out of its socket (glenoid cavity).

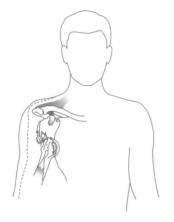

Shoulder dislocation: site of pain.

Loss of normal profile or appearance in the shoulder region.

Treatment

IMMEDIATE

Seek medical attention.

Place the arm in a sling for approximately ten days, making sure the elbow does not get stiff and the neck maintains a normal range of motion.

Practice isometric exercising the rotator cuff muscle while in a neutral joint position to help your range of flexibility.

Seek expert advice regarding your rehabilitation in order to prevent a recurrence of the dislocation.

If this is the first time you have dislocated your shoulder, relocation may occur itself.

LONG-TERM

Strengthen the muscle over a period of at least 6 to 12 weeks.

Don't expect full strength to return for six months or more.

Check range of movement in the muscle around the shoulder joint, to check for any muscle imbalances around the joint.

Respect the pain you are experiencing. You may have to limit the amount of sailing until your shoulder heals.

Follow the Pilates program outlined at the end of this chapter.

How to prevent

Don't hang on to the boom when sailing. Learn to release it in plenty of time.

Maintain good strength and good coordination in the shoulder and rotator cuff area (see page 101).

Biceps tendonitis

Biceps tendonitis is a common injury among athletes who use the majority of their upper body. The symptoms are very similar in appearance to impingement syndrome and the two conditions are often confused. Biceps tendonitis is a result of inflammation of the long head of the bicep at its insertion into the scapular (shoulder blade).

Pain tends to occur when the arm is lifted overhead and the elbow is flexed at greater than 90 degrees to the shoulder.

Causes

Poor technique or repetitive movement can cause this injury. Too much weight-pulling through the arm can exacerbate the problem because the tendon tends to become inflamed in the tendon groove.

Signs and symptoms

Tenderness in the front aspect of the shoulder joint (the biceps groove).

Pain when lifting the arm above the head.

Treatment

IMMEDIATE

Modify the amount of activity to avoid aggravating the pain.

Apply ice to the area.

LONG-TERM

Check the range of movement in the muscles around the shoulder joint. This determines whether there are any muscle imbalances around the joint.

Limit your sailing until you recover. Follow the Pilates recovery program outlined at the end of this chapter to expedite your recovery.

Check your overhead techniques when pulling the line in.

Low-back pain

Injuries to the spine are common in sailors and windsurfers, because of the constant bending required to lift, pull, or push.

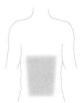

Low back pain affected area. Sailing may cause you to twist your back and cause injury to this area.

Causes

When sailing you may twist your back and remain like this for long periods of time. This can cause a muscle strain in the lower back area.

Signs and symptoms

Discomfort at the end of active movements such as forward bending, side bend or leaning backward.

Muscle tightness can be felt in the paravertebral muscle (the muscle on either side of the spine).

Nonspecific, low-back ache.

Treatment

IMMEDIATE

Take anti-inflammatories as prescribed by your medical practitioner.

Establish the contraction of the lower stomach muscle (transversus abdominis, see page 161).

Maintain the length in the hip flexor muscle (see page 74).

Assess your abdominal strength in order to determine the Pilates level you need to undertake to improve control and strength in your trunk. This is known as your dynamic core stability.

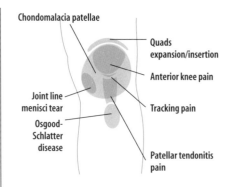

Sites of potential injury.

LONG-TERM

Improve the imbalance of your muscles in your spine: experiment with the range of motion in your spine and work on strengthening the weaker side to determine the direction of your limitations. (It may be advisable to have the muscle imbalance assessed properly by a chartered physiotherapist or osteopath).

Maintain the flexibility and strength to the lumbar spine. Follow the Pilates program at the end of this chapter.

Build your proprioception and reaction timing on a moving object (such as a wobble board) to improve your ability to move around a boat in a controlled and efficient manner. See page 13 for proprioception training.

PREVENTION

Build up the muscles you will need according to your role on the boat.

Improve your overall fitness level.

Patellofemoral pain

Patellofemoral pain occurs as a result of softening, and changes under the surface of the kneecap.

Causes

The main cause of a patellofemoral injury is through an imbalance in the quadriceps muscles. These muscles control the movement of the patella in the femoral groove.

Because of the "hiking out" position in dinghy sailing (hanging over the side of the boat to prevent it from capsizing) and keeping the knee in a semibent position, strain is placed on the quadriceps muscle group and kneecap.

Anterior knee pain because of variable exercises (see page 35 for anterior knee pain).

Overtraining, bending, squatting, and kneeling lead to the vastus medialis muscle wasting, leaving the patella to drift outward and cause friction against the outside of the femur bone at the knee joint (lateral femoral condyle).

Wasting of quadriceps.

Stress forms in the iliotibial band because of an imbalance in the tension along the band from the gluteus medius and minimus muscle and the tensor fasciae latae at the top of the band (gluteus medius/minimus). See page 44 for iliotibial band syndrome.

A hyper-extended knee (locking the knee backward).

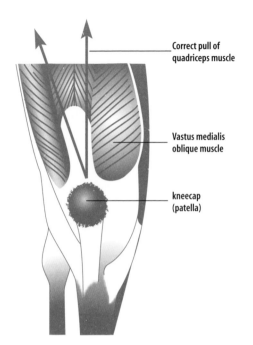

Correct pull of quadriceps muscle

Vastus medialis oblique muscle

kneecap (patella)

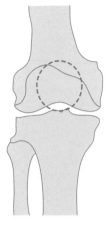

Ideal position of the kneecap within the knee joint.

Signs and symptoms

Tightness after sitting with bent knees for a period of time.

Excessive bending of the knees.

Patellofemoral crepitus and pain while contracting the quadriceps.

Pain when sailing or when in the hiking position.

Vague or nonspecific pain.

Tenderness on the medial side of patella.

Some swelling around the knee.

Legs giving away because of weakness in the quadriceps muscle.

Patellofemoral joint may be restricted during movement.

A wasting of the vastus medialis obliques (see diagram above).

Squatting will be painful.

To determine whether you have this condition, perform the Clarke's test on page 91.

Treatment

IMMEDIATE

P.R.I.C.E

Exercises for vastus medialis oblique (wall slides page 201, small knee bends in standing page 197). Taping to improve the tracking of the knee may be required. This needs to be applied by a medical practitioner.

LONG-TERM

Hip stabilization exercises (see page 175).

Maintain strength in the quadriceps

muscles, in particular the vastus medialis oblique (the muscle on the inside aspect of your knee).

Keep a good balance in the muscles by working on your single leg balance exercise (see page 178).

Maintain muscle control through the pelvis and pelvic stability (see page 175).

Ankle inversion injury

Ankle sprains are usually caused by the ankle rolling over and forcing the foot into dorsiflexion and inversion.

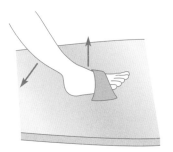

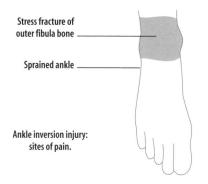

Stress fracture of outer fibula bone

Sprained ankle

Ankle inversion injury: sites of pain.

Causes

Landing awkwardly from a jump.

Changing direction suddenly.

Weak peroneal (ankle) muscles.

Tight Achilles tendon.

Existing ankle injury.

Signs and symptoms

Being able to pinpoint the exact location and feeling of the injury.

Feeling a popping sensation.

Feeling a tearing sensation, followed by a sharp pain.

The ankle is painful to touch.

Being unable to walk without feeling pain.

Swelling or bruising on the side of the foot.

Treatment

IMMEDIATE

Control pain and swelling through the following procedure:

P.R.I.C.E.

Bear weight only when tolerable.

Write the alphabet in the air with your foot to test the range of pain-free motion.

LONG-TERM

Achieve a good sense of balance with the ankle (see page 13).

Build strength around the ankle joint.

Be sensitive to pain when you feel it.

How to prevent

Maintain good strength and coordination around the ankle joint.

Follow the Pilates program on page 108 to improve your performance and prevent further ankle injuries.

Pilates exercises to improve performance and prevent further injury

▌ Lengthen
▼ Balance
● Strengthen

	Sailor's shoulder	Biceps tendonitis	Low-back pain	Patellofemoral pain	Ankle inversion injury	Shoulder dislocation
CORE EXERCISES						
curl up	●	●	●	●		●
diamond press	●	●				●
floating arms	●	●				●
four point challenge	▼	▼	▼			▼
hip opening			·		●	
pelvic stability			▌●	●	●	
neutral spine				●		
static standing balance				▼		
FOUNDATION EXERCISES						
arm circles	●	●				●
arm opening	▌	▌				▌
big squeeze			▌	●		
breathing patterns						
dart	▌●	▌●				▌●
hamstring lengthening				▌	●	
long sitting stretch	●	●		●	●	●
mid-back stretch		●				●
roll downs			●	▌	▌●	●
shoulder external rotation	●	●				●
shoulder internal rotation	●					●
shoulder push away		●				●
shoulder rotation control	▌	▌●				●
shoulder rowing	●	●				●
side reach	●	●	●	●		●
single knee kicks			●		▌●	
spinal curls			▌●		●	
standing squat				●	●	
star	●	●				●
T-band balance					▼	
threading the needle						
wall slides			●	●	▌●	
windows		●				

PERFORMANCE PILATES

	Sailor's shoulder	Biceps tendonitis	Low-back pain	Patellofemoral pain	Ankle inversion injury	Shoulder dislocation
bridging			●	●	●	
double leg stretch	■●	■	■	●		■●
hundred	●	●	●	●		●
lean forward bending			●	●	●	
leg pull prone	●	●	●			●
leg pull back			●			
lunge			●	●	●	
mermaid	●		●			●
oblique curl up			●			
open leg rocker			■●	●		
Pilates push up	●	●				▼●
praying mantis	●	●	●			
roll up					■	
rolling like a ball			■			
scissors			■●	●		
shoulder challenge	●	●				●
side kick series				●	■●	
side rolls			●			
single leg stretch			■	●	■●	
sitting knee folds			●			
superman	●	●				●
swimming	●	●	■●	■●	■	●
teaser			●			
tennis ball raises				●	■●	
torpedo	●	●		●		●
waist twists in standing			■●			

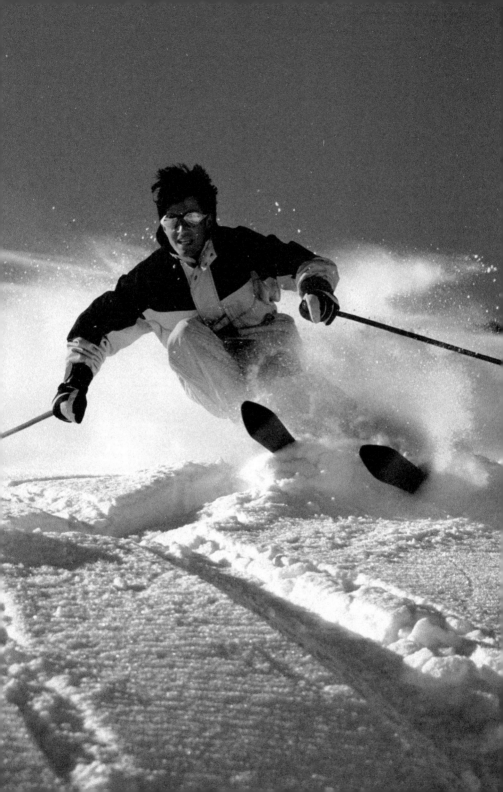

Skiing and Snowboarding

Skiing is fast growing as the most popular family sport. While it is relatively safe, injuries do occur. If you are a beginner, it is three to five times more likely that you will be injured on the slope than competent skiers. Women and children may be at slightly higher risk to overall injury than men. However, because of the high speeds at which most men ski, men are more likely to suffer from severe knee sprain and muscle fatigue. Also, men, particularly in the twenty-to-thirty age group, sustain more serious head and neck injuries than are sustained by women.

Common skiing injuries

Neck sprain

A sprain is a tear in a muscle or tendon. Your neck is surrounded by small muscles, which run close to the vertebrae, and larger muscles, which make up the visible muscles of the neck. Neck sprains most often occur when the head and neck are forcibly moved, such as in a whiplash injury or from contact in sport. When skiing, a neck-sprain injury can range from a minor bump on the head to life threatening trauma, depending on the force of impact and area of head injury.

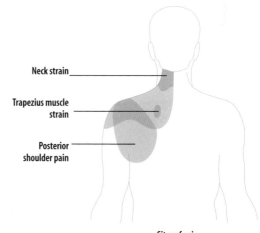

Neck strain

Trapezius muscle strain

Posterior shoulder pain

Sites of pain.

111

Shoulder injuries

Causes

There are several types of shoulder injuries that can occur when skiing:

Fractured clavicle: caused by falling onto your outstretched arm. The force of impact travels up the arm to the collarbone.

Fractured humerus: caused by falling directly onto the upper part of the arm.

Falling onto the shoulder/collarbone.

Signs and symptoms

Tenderness at top of the shoulder bone.

Pain on movement, particularly when you reach across toward the opposite shoulder.

Treatment

IMMEDIATE

Apply ice to the area for ten minutes or until the area is numb.

The arm will need to be supported to help reduce pain. Use a sling.

LONG-TERM

Tape the area to provide support while skiing.

Undertake a comprehensive Pilates program for the shoulder area. See the Pilates program at the end of this chapter.

Shoulder dislocation

A shoulder dislocation is when the top part of the arm bone (humeral head) slips out of its socket (glenoid cavity). Forward (anterior) dislocations are most common. When this occurs the anterior inferior

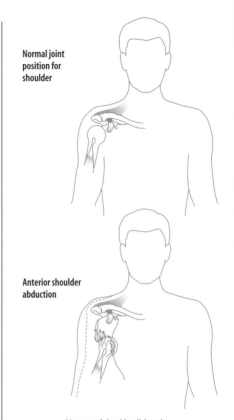

Normal joint position for shoulder

Anterior shoulder abduction

Diagram of shoulder dislocation.

labrum (a piece of cartilage that stabilizes the shoulder) frequently is torn. Shoulder dislocations can also occur backward (posterior) and downward (inferior). Repeated dislocations and multidirectional shoulder instability are also possible.

Causes

A dislocation can occur when the arm is forcibly moved into an awkward position during a fall. If a dislocation or partial dislocation (known as a subluxation) occurs from only a minor amount of force, recurrent or multidirectional instability must be considered.

Signs and symptoms

Loss of active range of movement in the shoulder joint in most directions.

Feeling the joint "pop out."

Loss of normal profile or appearance in the shoulder region.

Treatment

IMMEDIATE

If this is the first time you have dislocated your shoulder, the relocation may occur by itself. Nevertheless, medical attention is required.

Place the arm in a sling for approximately ten days, making sure the elbow does not get stiff and the neck maintains a normal range of motion.

Practice isometric exercises using the rotator cuff muscles while in a neutral joint position to help your range of flexibility.

Seek expert advice regarding rehabilitation in order to prevent the injury occurring again.

LONG-TERM

Strengthening the muscle will take at least 6 to 12 weeks.

Don't expect full strength to return for six months or more.

Check range of movement in the muscle around the shoulder joint, to determine whether or not there are any muscle imbalances around the joint.

Respect the pain you are experiencing. You may have to limit the amount of skiing you do until your shoulder heals.

How to prevent

Don't hang on to your poles when skiing. Learn to release them in plenty of time.

Maintain good strength and coordination to the shoulder and rotator cuff area (see page 25).

Medial ligament injury

Causes

Forcing the knee into a gaping position on the inside of the knee.

Losing control and falling when traveling at high speed.

The binding of the ski doesn't release the foot when you fall. As a result, the knee becomes twisted, placing a force on the knee ligament and creating a tear.

Signs and symptoms

Pain on the inside of the knee. The amount of pain will determine the degree of injury present.

Swelling in the knee area.

Pain when skiing, particularly when attempting a sudden change in direction.

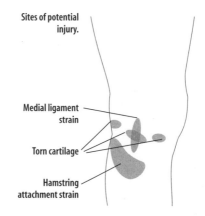

Sites of potential injury.

Medial ligament strain

Torn cartilage

Hamstring attachment strain

Tenderness along the length of the ligament.

Treatment
IMMEDIATE

P.R.I.C.E. Control swelling with the application of ice for ten minutes or until the area is numb.

Protect the ligament from further damage: wear a brace or tape the knee.

LONG-TERM

Reduce or minimize the swelling by applying ice for ten minutes, or until the area is numb. Apply every two hours.

Build up support of quadriceps muscles.

Maintain a general level of fitness, through aqua jogging—or cycling—as long as the pain is minimal.

Participate in activities that build up your lower-limb balance and coordination of movement.

Anterior cruciate ligament injury

The knee has four ligaments holding it in place: one at each side to stop the bones sliding sideways and two crossing over in the middle to stop the bones sliding forward and backward. The latter two, in the middle, are called the cruciate ligaments. They are the posterior cruciate ligament (at the back) and anterior cruciate ligament (at the front). If these are damaged in any way they may cause knee pain. The main job of the anterior cruciate ligament in the knee is passively to stabilize the knee and supply sensory information to the central nervous system.

Causes
The ligament can be injured by twisting the knee or because of an impact to the side of the knee—often the outside.

Signs and symptoms
Gradual swelling of the knee area. If the swelling takes place over a period of two hours, this can indicate a small amount of damage to the soft tissue.

The sensation of the knee separating or a "gapping" when the injury occurs. This is a result of a tear in the ligament.

Severe pain when the injury occurs. It's unlikely you'll be able to continue playing. This pain may dissipate quickly and you'll be able to move your knee forward, but any twisting movement will cause pain again. This is because of the instability of the knee stabilizers.

Use the anterior draw test (see opposite) to determine extent of injury.

Treatment
IMMEDIATE

Control the swelling through the use of P.R.I.C.E. compression on the knee area. Ice will help reduce the amount of pain.

LONG-TERM

The extent of the injury is determined by the degree of damage to the ligament. Complete or partial rupture may require repair or reconstruction. It will need to be assessed by a medical practitioner.

If the ligament has been stretched and not torn (there will be a minimal amount of swelling and anterior draw test will fail), follow the treatment plan for knee ligaments on page 123.

Ligament damage to the knee.

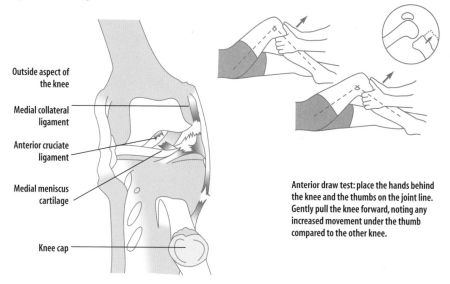

Outside aspect of the knee

Medial collateral ligament

Anterior cruciate ligament

Medial meniscus cartilage

Knee cap

Anterior draw test: place the hands behind the knee and the thumbs on the joint line. Gently pull the knee forward, noting any increased movement under the thumb compared to the other knee.

How to prevent

To reduce the swelling, every two hours apply ice for ten minutes or until the area is numb.

Build up the support of the quadriceps muscles.

Maintain a general level of fitness through aqua jogging, cycling, or walking. These exercises should keep pain to a minimum.

Follow the Pilates program at the end of this chapter to help improve lower-limb balance, coordination, and endurance.

Common snowboarding injuries

Snowboarding, a winter sport that has almost overtaken skiing in popularity, requires strength, agility, and flexible joints. As both feet are strapped onto the snowboard and always face the same direction, it's important to keep the knees static and to prevent them from twisting. Most injuries in snowboarding occur in the upper body, as this area usually takes the full force of a fall.

Wrist injury

Injuries tend to occur to the leading hand and wrist, as it's common to use your favored hand to break your fall.
Because of the force of impact, injuries can also occur in the shoulder tissue, back and head.

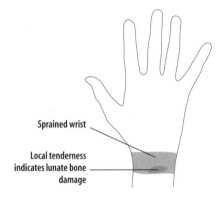

Sprained wrist

Local tenderness indicates lunate bone damage

Causes

Injury to the wrist area can be caused by falling onto your outstretched arm, forcing the wrist into an unnatural extension. Consequently, this can damage the delicate tendons and muscles of the wrist area.

Signs and symptoms

Tenderness in the wrist area, particularly in the soft tissue.

The wrist can still be moved, but with some pain.

Treatment

IMMEDIATE

Use the P.R.I.C.E. method, according to the level of pain.

Tape the wrist to prevent it being forced backward.

Exercise the muscle on either side of the wrist joint. This helps to build up the muscles which act as a dynamic brace to prevent further injury.

Move your fingers, while keeping your wrist neutral (see page 233 for wrist strengthening exercise).

LONG-TERM

If it is a subluxed joint—too much movement in the joint in its normal position—you will need to build the dynamic support.

Exercise

Open and close your fingers several times. Keep your wrist in a straight line with the forearm. As your strength and flexibility increases, build up the speed of the movement. Grip a stress ball to make the exercise more effective.

How to prevent

When you fall, try to tuck your arm into your side, with your fists clenched.

Wear a wrist protector. Choose from either a stand alone wrist guard, or an integrated glove/guard system.

Improve your static standing balance by working on your trunk control and core stability (see page 160).

Ankle injuries

It is extremely common to suffer from snowboarder's ankle: a fracture of the talus bone (the main bone in the central aspect of the ankle).

Sites of pain.

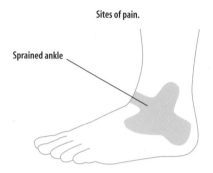

Sprained ankle

Causes

Fractures to this area occur as a result of forced dorsiflexion and foot inversion— where the foot is pulled upward and the sole of the foot is twisted inward.

Landing on the foot awkwardly.

Signs and symptoms

You are able to describe the actual mechanism of injury.

The ankle is painful to touch, even at rest.

You are unable to walk without pain.

There is swelling and bruising on the side of the foot.

Signs and symptoms are similar to inversion injuries of the ankle.

Treatment

IMMEDIATE

Control pain and swelling through P.R.I.C.E. for the first three days.

Practice range of motion exercises. Write the alphabet in the air with your foot, within the pain-free range.

Tape the joint for at least seven days to protect any further damage occurring.

Bear weight as tolerable.

Phases of care

PHASE ONE

Apply P.R.I.C.E. until the swelling has reduced and the ankle is able to bear your full body-weight.

PHASE TWO

Restore normal range of motion and strength to the ankle joint. It may be useful to wear a brace to help control the range of movement.

PHASE THREE

Begin this phase when the range of movement is almost normal and the pain and the swelling have disappeared.

Restore the coordination of movements required for snowboarding.

LONG-TERM

If the fracture is not recognized or treated, this can lead to the bones failing to knit evenly together and a severe degeneration of the sub-talar joint.

Use a non-weight-bearing brace for about four weeks. Following this, use a walking cast for two weeks.

Joint mobilization will be required when the cast is removed, because the ankle will be stiff.

Follow the Pilates program outlined at the end of the chapter.

Pilates exercises to improve performance and prevent further injury

I   Lengthen
▼   Balance
●   Strengthen

	Neck strain	Shoulder injuries	Shoulder dislocation	Medial ligament injury	Anterior cruciate ligament injury
CORE EXERCISES					
curl up	●	●			
diamond press	●	●	●		
floating arms	●	●	●		
four point challenge	▼	▼	▼		
hip opening				●	●
pelvic stability				●	●
static standing balance				▼	▼
FOUNDATION EXERCISES					
arm circles		●	●		
arm opening	●	I	I		
dart	●	I●	I●		
hamstring lengthening				I	I
long sitting stretch		●	●	●	●
mid-back stretch	●	●	●		
neck rolls	●				
roll downs	I	●	●		
shoulder external rotation		●	●		
shoulder internal rotation		●	●		
shoulder push away		●	●		
shoulder rowing		●			
shoulder rotation control	●	I			
side reach	●	●	●		
single knee kick				I●	I●
spinal curls				●	●
standing squat				●	●
star	●	●	●	●	●

	Neck strain	Shoulder injuries	Shoulder dislocation	Medial ligament injury	Anterior cruciate ligament injury
T-band balance				▼	▼
threading the needle	●				
wall slides	▮			●	●
windows	●	●	●		
PERFORMANCE PILATES					
bridging				●	●
double leg stretch	●	▮ ●	▮ ●		
eccentric hamstrings				●	●
hundred	●	●	●		
knee/leg circles				●	●
leg pull prone	●	●	●	●	●
leg pull back	●			●	●
mermaid		●	●		
open leg rocker				▮ ●	▮ ●
Pilates push up	●	▼ ●	▼ ●		
praying mantis	●	●	●	●	●
scissors				●	●
shoulder challenge		●	●		
side rolls				●	●
single leg stretch	●			●	●
sitting knee folds				●	●
superman		●	●		
swimming	●	●	●	▮ ●	▮ ●
teaser	●				
tennis ball raises				●	●
torpedo		●	●	●	●

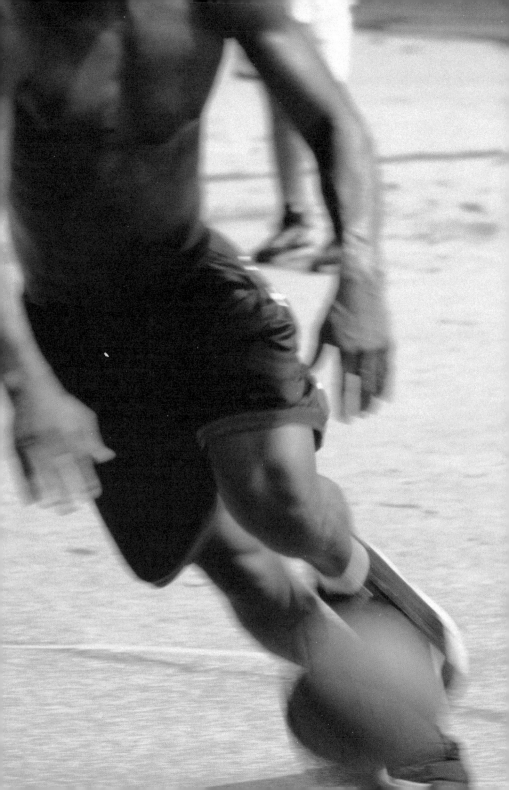

Soccer

Soccer is a rigorous sport that demands rapid speed changes, pivoting, sideways and backward displacement, and jumping motions that combine all these movements. Thus it is inevitable that soccer players are predisposed to injury. Soccer injuries that respond to Pilates treatment are those affecting the lower limbs. Injuries to the upper leg often result from direct blows and can lead to bruising in the muscle area. Injuries sustained around the knee, usually because of twisting actions or blows to the knee, tend to place stress on the ligament. Wearing the correct studs in your shoes and using shin pads are important to prevent severe injuries in the lower limbs.

Common soccer injuries

Acromioclavicular joint sprain

The acromioclavicular (AC) joint sits between the outside end of the clavicle and part of the shoulder blade (the acromion). A ligament connects the two and holds the joint together. A fall directly on the outside of the upper arm may lead to the ligament being damaged and torn, and can distort the joint.

Causes

AC sprains may be caused by falling backward while throwing the ball in from the sideline. The arm needs to be highly extended or in abduction or an external rotation position for the sprain to occur.

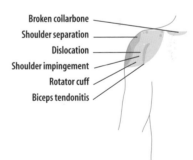

Broken collarbone
Shoulder separation
Dislocation
Shoulder impingement
Rotator cuff
Biceps tendonitis

Diagram of affected area: sites of pain.

Signs and symptoms

Pain, tenderness, or possible deformity around the AC .

Classification of pain

GRADE ONE PAIN

Symptoms: Pain or tenderness.

Treatment: Treat symptoms through P.R.I.C.E. Continue activity.

GRADE TWO PAIN

Symptoms: Pain, tenderness, and slight separation from the prominent end of the clavicle.

Treatment: Use a sling and rest for two to four weeks depending on severity.

GRADE THREE PAIN

Symptoms: Pain, tenderness, and marked separation of the joint with a prominent end of the clavicle.

Treatment: You may need to wear a brace and rest for six to eight weeks. Surgery may be necessary.

Groin injuries

Soccer involves kicking the ball and a fair amount of power, so the groin is vulnerable to injury owing to the sudden overstretching of the leg and thigh muscles. As the leg tends to turn outward during a kicking action, its muscles are put under strain.

Causes

Forces involved in the kick (opposing force, full swing, or sudden impact with the ground) may overstretch the muscle fibers and the bony tissue of the pelvic ring and pubic sympnysis (the joint in the center of the pelvis). Overusing the adductor muscles or over training can also lead to injury.

Signs and symptoms

Tightening of the groin muscles. Pain may

Adductor muscles: sites of pain.

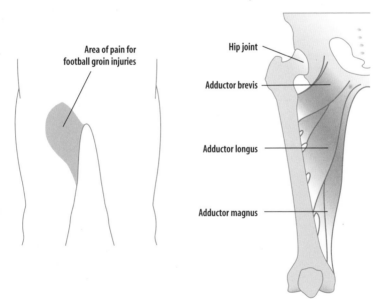

Area of pain for
football groin injuries

Hip joint

Adductor brevis

Adductor longus

Adductor magnus

not be present until the day after the game.

A sudden sharp pain in the groin and/or adductor muscles.

Bruising or swelling around the groin area, which may occur afterward.

Inability to contract adductor muscles.

A lump or gap in the adductor muscles.

Treatment
IMMEDIATE

Reduce bruising and swelling. Use the P.R.I.C.E application.

Stretch gently.

Do not use strengthening exercises for at least four days (see page 130).

Achieve a passive range of motion before progressing to stretching. Gradually increase the range of strengthening as bearable.

LONG-TERM

Gradually increase the intensity of the stretch, increasing the range of movement (see knee folds page 175).

Maintain the pelvis in a neutral spine position (see page 177).

Recurrent strain is caused by poor rehabilitation in the early stages of injury or by returning to sport too quickly. This may be as a result of stiffness in the lumbar spine area.

How to prevent

Maintain passive range and strength of the groin muscles (see the strengthening exercises at the end of the chapter).

If the problem is recurrent you will need to get the groin injury assessed properly by a medical practitioner.

Knee injuries

During a soccer game the knee is put under large amounts of strain. It is reported to be the most serious site of injury. The injuries are caused by collisions, sudden twisting and direct impacts on the side of the knee.

Knee injuries can occur when the two collateral ligaments (medial and lateral ligaments) are damaged. The medial ligament is on the inside of the knee. The lateral ligament is on the outside of the knee and is meant to prevent the joint from gaping.

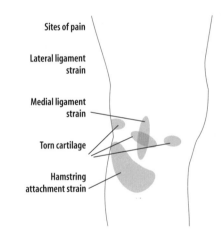

Sites of pain

Lateral ligament strain

Medial ligament strain

Torn cartilage

Hamstring attachment strain

Medial ligament injury

Causes

Forcing the knee into a gaping position on the inside of the knee.

The knee is suddenly twisted, with the foot fixed on the ground, possibly owing to the studs of the shoe.

Signs and symptoms

Pain on the inside of the knee. The amount of pain will determine the degree of injury present.

Swelling in the knee area.

Tenderness along the length of the ligament.

Pain when running, particularly when attempting a sudden change in direction.

Discomfort when kicking the ball using the inside of the foot.

Treatment

IMMEDIATE

P.R.I.C.E. Control swelling with the application of ice for ten minutes or until the area is numb.

Protect the ligament from further damage: wear a brace or tape the knee.

LONG-TERM

Reduce or minimize the swelling by applying ice for ten minutes, or until the area is numb. Apply every two hours.

Build up support of quadriceps muscles.

Maintain a general level of fitness, through aqua jogging—or cycling—as long as the pain is minimal.

Participate in activities that build up your lower-limb balance and coordination of movement.

Anterior cruciate ligament injury

The knee has four ligaments holding it in place: one at each side to stop the bones sliding sideways and two crossing over in the middle to stop the bones sliding forward and backward. The latter two, in

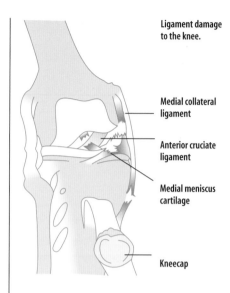

Ligament damage to the knee.

Medial collateral ligament

Anterior cruciate ligament

Medial meniscus cartilage

Kneecap

the middle, are called the cruciate ligaments. They are the posterior cruciate ligament (at the back) and anterior cruciate ligament (at the front). If these are damaged in any way they may cause knee pain. The main job of the anterior cruciate ligament in the knee is passively to stabilize the knee and supply sensory information to the central nervous system.

Causes

The ligament can be injured by twisting the knee or because an impact to the side of the knee—often the outside.

Signs and symptoms

Gradual swelling of the knee area. If the swelling takes place over a period of two hours, this can indicate a small amount of damage to the soft tissue.

The sensation of the knee separating or a

"gapping" when the injury occurs. This is a result of a tear in the ligament.

Severe pain when the injury occurs. It's unlikely you'll be able to continue playing. This pain may dissipate quickly and you'll be able to move your knee forward, but any twisting movement will cause pain again. This is because of the instability of the knee stabilizers.

Use the anterior draw test (below) to determine the extent of the injury.

Treatment

IMMEDIATE

Control the swelling through the use of P.R.I.C.E. compression on the knee area.

Ice will help reduce the amount of pain.

LONG-TERM

The extent of the injury is determined by the degree of damage to the ligament. Complete or partial rupture may require repair or reconstruction. It will need to be assessed by a medical practitioner.

If the ligament has been stretched and

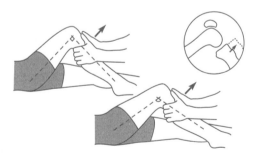

Anterior draw test: place the hands behind the knee and the thumbs on the joint line. Gently pull the knee forward. Noting any increase movement under the thumb when compared with the other knee will indicate the presence of increased movement.

not torn (there will be a minimal amount of swelling and Anterior draw test will fail), follow the treatment plan for knee ligaments on page 126.

How to prevent

To reduce the swelling, every two hours apply ice for ten minutes or until the area is numb.

Build up the support of the quadriceps muscles.

Maintain a general level of fitness through aqua jogging, cycling, or walking. These exercises should keep pain to a minimum.

Follow a program to help improve lower-limb balance, coordination, and endurance.

Meniscus tear

There are two menisci in your knee which rest between the thigh bone (femur) and shin bone (tibia). One meniscus rests on the medial tibial plateau; this is the medial meniscus. The other meniscus rests on the lateral tibial plateau—the lateral meniscus. The meniscus' main function is to distribute the weight evenly in the leg, to prevent any damage to the knee joint.

The most common traumatic meniscus tear occurs when the knee joint is bent (flexed) and the knee is then twisted. It is not uncommon for the meniscus tear to occur along with injuries to the anterior cruciate ligament and the medial collateral ligament. When all three occur together they are known as the "unhappy triad,"

Types of meniscus tears

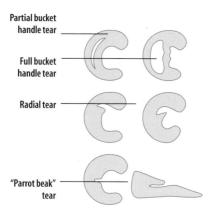

Partial bucket handle tear

Full bucket handle tear

Radial tear

"Parrot beak" tear

Treatment

CONSERVATIVE

Symptoms develop over 24 hours.

There is minimal swelling.

There is full range of movement, with pain only at end of range.

Pain during McMurray test in the inner range of flexion.

Surgery may be required if:

Injury is due to severe twisting motion.

Player is unable to continue.

Knee clicks during McMurray test.

Tear associated with anterior cruciate ligament.

Little improvement after three weeks of ongoing treatment.

which may happen in sports such as soccer when the player is hit on the outside of the knee.

Causes

Twisting the knee while the foot is anchored to the ground.

Progressive wear on the whole joint (often found in people over 40).

Signs and symptoms

Swelling proportional to activity.

Pain on rotation or flexion.

Pain on joint line.

Feeling of weakness and insecurity in the legs, or the knee actually giving way.

Locking sensation in the knee.

Generalized ache in the knee.

Positive McMurray test (see right).

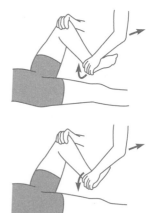

Mc Murray test: Lie down and bend your injured knee. Ask a partner to put one hand over your knee, while supporting your heel with the other hand. Pulling up on your heel, they should gently turn your knee outward and straighten your leg (keeping your knee turned out). Bend your leg again and this time rotate the knee inward by pressing around the heel, and then straighten the leg. Pain in achieving a straight leg indicates a positive result.

Treatment

IMMEDIATE

Control swelling through P.R.I.C.E.

Maintain an active range of motion.

Maintain a contraction of the quadriceps for the count of three, then release.

LONG-TERM

Keep swelling to a minimum by applying ice regularly after exercise if pain continues.

Continue stretching to maintain a full range of movement.

Follow the Pilates program at the end of this chapter.

How to prevent

Train all-year round to ensure you are fit enough for the soccer season. This will help prevent muscle injuries.

Follow the Pilates flexibility program at the end of this chapter.

Strengthen the particular muscles used during a match: neck, abdominals, and the trunk.

Always warm up before starting a game.

Shin splints

Shin splints is a term commonly used to describe lower leg pains that are non-specific in nature. In soccer, the most common injuries are caused by kicks to the shin during a tackle. Bruising can be severe and a fracture can be sustained on the front of the leg, particularly the fibula.

Components of shin splints:

1. Bone stress, leading to a fracture.

2. Inflammation at the insertion of the muscles in the compartments of the lower leg.

3. Raised intracompartment pressure. Each muscle compartment is covered in thick inelastic fascia. If muscles are overused they will become inflamed and extremely painful.

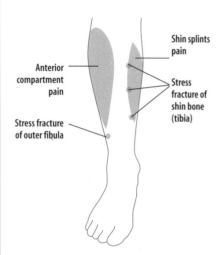

Anterior compartment pain

Stress fracture of outer fibula

Shin splints pain

Stress fracture of shin bone (tibia)

Diagram of affected area: sites of pain.

Main areas of shin pain

Type of pain: localized, acute, or sharp.

Factors: constant or increasing pain that becomes worse on impact.

Other symptoms: night ache that increases in the morning.

Caused by: sudden increase in training. Muscle fatigue leading to bone loading. Inadequate footwear to support the feet while running.

Area: **muscle inflammation**

Type of pain: Inside border of the tibia.

Factors: Pain decreases after warming up.

Other symptoms: Worst in the morning and after exercising.

Caused by: Training on hard surfaces. Increasing exercise intensity too rapidly. Poor biomechanics during running. Repetitive jumping.

Area: **compartment syndrome**

Type of pain: Aching tightness known as intermittent claudication pain during activity and afterward.

Factors: Increases with exercise. Decreases with rest.

Other symptoms: At worst muscle weakness.

Caused by: Sudden increase in exercise intensity. Prolonged exercise bouts.

Treatment

IMMEDIATE

Treat the pain as early as possible.

Apply ice to the tender area, moving it around the area for up to ten minutes.

Rest for two to three weeks. When you begin training again, change your training onto an even surface.

Make sure you have the right footwear for your training (see page 16).

If your muscles are inflamed, follow a specific stretching program.

How to prevent

Wear shin pads for protection.

Wear the correct footwear for training.

Warm up completely before playing.

Concentrate on flexing your muscles, especially lower limbs during warm up.

Ankle inversion injury

Ankle sprains are by far the most common injuries in sports. They're usually caused by the ankle rolling over and the foot is forced into dorsiflexion and inversion.

Causes

Landing awkwardly from a jump.

Stepping or landing on an opponent's foot.

Changing direction suddenly.

Sudden deceleration during a run.

Running on an uneven surface.

Weak peroneal (ankle) muscles.

Tight Achilles tendon.

Previous ankle injury.

Signs and symptoms

Being able to pinpoint the exact location and feeling of the injury.

Feeling a popping sensation.

Feeling a tearing sensation, followed by sharp pain.

Painful to touch.

Unable to walk without feeling pain.

Swelling or bruising on side of the foot.

Treatment

IMMEDIATE

Control the pain and swelling through the following procedures:

P.R.I.C.E.

Place weight on the ankle only when it is bearable.

Write the alphabet in the air with your foot to test the range of pain-free motion.

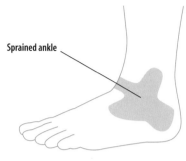

Sprained ankle

Sprained ankle: site of pain.

LONG-TERM

Achieve a good sense of balance with the ankle.

Build strength around the ankle joint.

Be sensitive to pain when you feel it.

How to prevent

Maintain good strength and coordination around the ankle joint.

Follow the exercise program at the end of this chapter to improve your performance and prevent further ankle injuries.

Soccer ankle

Soccer ankle is defined by chronic ankle pain following previous ankle sprains. This can be because of an irritation to the outer layer of the bone (chronic periostitis) on the anterior margin of the lower end of the tibia and over the talus.

Causes

Repeatedly kicking the ball with the top and inside of the foot.

Signs and symptoms

Pain when kicking a ball or lunging.

Stiffness or soreness at the end of the joint.

Lack of speed at the beginning of a run.

Treatment

IMMEDIATE

Control the pain and swelling by applying P.R.I.C.E. for the first three days.

Bear weight as tolerable.

Write the alphabet in the air with your foot to test your pain-free range.

Tape the joint for at least seven days to prevent it from further damage.

LONG-TERM

Apply P.R.I.C.E. until you are able to bear your weight comfortably and the swelling is reduced.

Focus on restoring a normal range of motion and strength in the joint. When your range of motion is nearly returned and pain and swelling is absent, wear a brace to help control range of motion.

Improve on your coordination.

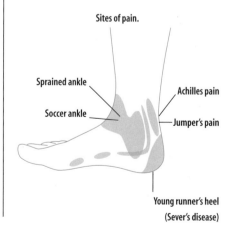

Sites of pain.

Sprained ankle

Soccer ankle

Achilles pain

Jumper's pain

Young runner's heel
(Sever's disease)

Pilates exercises to improve performance and prevent further injury

❙ Lengthen
▼ Balance
● Strengthen

	Acromioclavicular sprain	Groin injuries	Medial ligament strain	Anterior cruciate ligament strain	Meniscus tear	Shin splints	Ankle inversion injury	Soccer ankle
CORE EXERCISES								
curl up	●	●	●	●			●	
hip opening	●	●	●	●	●	●	●	●
pelvic stability	❙●	●	●	●	●	●	●	
neutral spine	●							
static standing balance	▼	●▼	▼	▼	▼	▼	▼	▼
FOUNDATION EXERCISES								
hamstring lengthening	❙		❙	❙	❙			
long sitting stretch		●	●	●	●	●	●	●
roll downs	❙●			●		❙	❙●	❙
side reach	●			●				
single knee kicks		❙		❙●	❙	❙	●	❙●
spinal curls	❙●	●	●			●	●	
standing squat	●	●	●		●	●	●	
star	●	●						
T-band balance	▼	▼		▼	▼	▼	▼	▼
wall slides						●	❙	❙●	❙

PERFORMANCE PILATES	Acromioclavicular sprain	Groin injuries	Medial ligament strain	Anterior cruciate ligament strain	Meniscus tear	Shin splints	Ankle inversion injury	Soccer ankle
bridging			●	●	●		●	
double leg stretch		▮						
eccentric hamstrings				●		●		
heel drop		●				●		●
hundred		●						
knee circles			▮ ●	▮ ●			▮	▮
lean forward standing		●				●	●	
leg pull back				●				
leg pull prone			●	●	●			
lunge						●	●	●
oblique curl ups		●						
open leg rocker		●	▮ ●	●	●			
praying mantis				●				
roll up					●	●		
rolling like a ball		▮			●			
scissors		▮ ●	●	●	●			
side kick series		▮ ●				●	●	●
side rolls		▮	●					
single leg stretch		▮ ●	●	●		●	●	
sitting knee folds			●	●	●			
swimming		●	▮ ●	▮ ●	●	●		
tennis ball raises		●	●	●	●	●	●	● ●
torpedo		●	●	●				

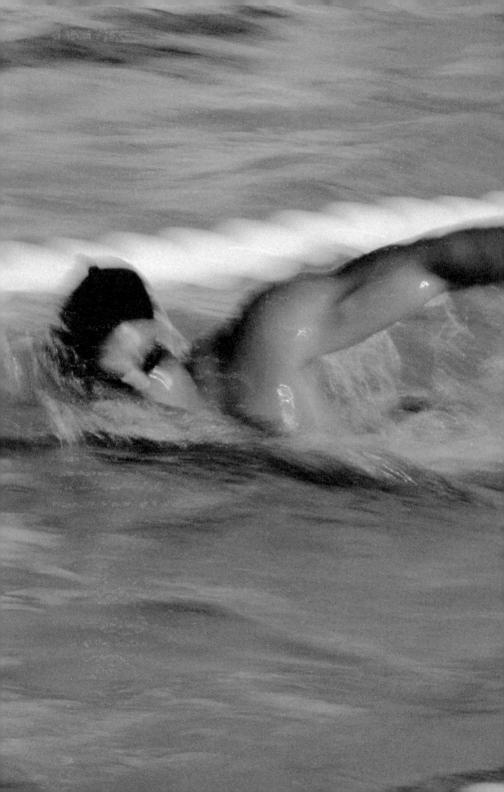

Swimming

Swimming has a low incidence of serious injuries due to the lack of force or strain on the muscles. Problems tend to arise only because of overtraining or overuse. Swimming injuries mainly occur in the shoulders, back, and knees. Shoulder injuries relate to the repetitive and high-speed movement of the rotating arms and the effort involved in controlling your position in the water. Problems arise through an imbalance of muscles or an inflammation of the muscles around the shoulder joint. These injuries can cause pain and limit the ability to swim effectively. Pain to the knee area is usually associated with the breaststroke kicking action—incorrect kicking action can place strain on the ligaments.

Common swimming injuries

Swimmer's shoulder

There are three main reasons why swimming can cause shoulder injuries:

1. Excessive movement of the shoulder joint in the joint capsule.

2. Impingement problems because of the mechanical obstruction of the rotator cuff tendons under the anterior inferior of the acromion and associated loss of space in the subacromial area.

3. Muscle imbalance—as a result of changes to muscle length and strength around the shoulder and shoulder blade.

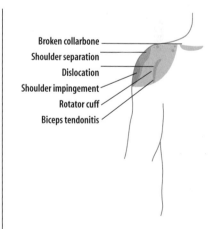

Broken collarbone
Shoulder separation
Dislocation
Shoulder impingement
Rotator cuff
Biceps tendonitis

Rotator cuff area: sites of pain.

Causes

Weakness of the muscle at the back of the shoulder joint (posterior deltoid/infraspinatus/teres minor).

Too much external rotation of the actual shoulder joint into external rotation.

Identify the painful phase of the stroke to help determine the structures involved.

Signs and symptoms

Rate your pain between one and six:

1-2 Continue swimming. Use local ice application.

3-4 Modify training.

5-6 Seek comprehensive assessment and stop training.

Visual assessment

Postural alignment

A typical swimmer's posture—rounded shoulders and protracted shoulder blade—can lead to a muscle imbalance. This is where the anterior chest muscles shorten and weaken the posterior shoulder and, in turn, shoulder-blade muscles.

Scapulohumeral rhythm

This is where the shoulder moves on the shoulder blade. A normal movement is two degrees of movement in the arm to one degree of movement in the shoulder blade. If this area moves, it indicates a loss of this balance. Do the floating arm exercise (see page 172). This will help identify the changes to the rhythm between the arm movement and the balance of the shoulder blade.

Scapula and humerus movement is a finely tuned balance of mobility and stability.

Range of motion

Loss of range may indicate tightness of muscle units (see imbalance chart on page 141).

Muscle imbalance

Signs and symptoms

Postural deformities of rounded shoulders and thoracic kyphosis.

Weakness of the posterior rotator cuff muscles and shoulder blade stabilizer muscles.

Limited internal rotation of the shoulder joint and excessive external rotation of the shoulder. Decay of normal scapulo-humeral rhythm.

How to prevent

Maintain a balance between the length of the internal rotators (teres major, subscapularis) and the external rotators (teres minor and infraspinatus). See shoulder rotation exercise (page 192).

Take swimming lessons. The teacher will observe your stroke and assess any imbalances.

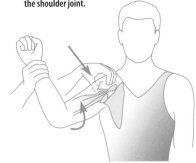

Apprehension test: pressure on the back of the shoulder results in pain indicating instability in the shoulder joint.

Free-style stroke action

RECOVERY PHASE

PULL THROUGH

PULL THROUGH

Stage:	Shoulder action	Muscles involved
Hand entry	Abductor/external rotation	Serratus anterior, subscapularis
Mid-pull-through	90-degree abduction Neutral rotation	Pectoralis major, teres minor, Subscapularis, biceps, latissimus dorsi/deltoid, upper trapezius
End of pull-through	Abduction/internal rotation	Rhomboid, supraspinatus, deltoid, serratus anterior

RECOVERY PHASE

Elbow lift	Adductor/ internal rotation	mid deltoid, supraspinatus
Mid recovery	90-degree external rotation	infraspinatus, subscapularis,
Hand entry	Abductor/internal rotation	infraspinatus

Evaluating your swimming stroke

Check to make sure your elbows don't drop during late recovery stage. This indicates early fatigue in the shoulder muscles leading to impingement.

Check to see how much your body rolls when swimming. It shouldn't roll more than 40 degrees.

If your head is too low, this can place strain on your arm.

If your head is too high in the water it can increase the amount of body drag.

Breathe from both sides. Breathing only on one side can increase problems on the opposite side.

Keep your kicks even. This will help to keep your movements streamlined and steady.

Presence of arc pain indicates possible shoulder impingement.

Shoulder impingement

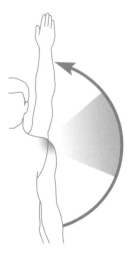

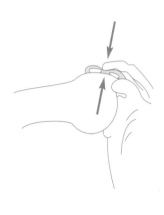

Avoid overtraining to reduce muscle fatigue in the shoulder joint and/or shoulder blade.

Training regime

Gradually increase distance and intensity. Do the vigorous laps at the beginning.

Make sure you do a proper warm-up and cool-down.

Strengthening

Include external rotator exercises (see page 189) in dry-land sessions. Practice more than three times a week.

Stretching

Make sure that there is no pain involved.

Treatment

IMMEDIATE

Determine the cause of the shoulder problem in order to modify the aggravating factors.

Increasing your flexibility for swimming

Muscle: *Pectoralis major/minor*

Exercise: **Arm opening** (page 180) **double leg stretch with your feet down** (page 205)

Muscle: *Trapezius*

Exercise: **Mid-back stretch** (page 186)

Muscle: *Biceps*

Exercise: **Dart** (page 183)

Muscle: *Triceps*

Exercise: **Diamond press** (page 170)

Muscle: *Serratus anterior*

Exercise: **Four point challenge** (page 170), **Pilates push up** (page 217)

Muscle: *Subscapularis*

Exercise: **shoulder rotation** (page 192)

Sports specific

Stroke changes reduce distance swimming.

Stroke mechanics:

limit extremes of abduction/internal rotation by keeping elbows high, and not reaching too far forward.

Swimming equipment:

Use a standard-sized kickboard, due to position of the shoulder in impingement aim above head. As big floating kickboards push shoulders up under the acromial joint.

Limit use hand paddles, cause stress in the pull through muscles. Good, easy warm up /swim down.

Use of swim fins in early stage enables swimmers to train with speed using a strong kick. This reduces strain on the shoulder muscles.

Apply ice to the front of the shoulder joints, for ten minutes, or until the area is numb.

Use anti-inflammatories as directed.

Physiotherapy modalities—local joint mobilization techniques.

Practice isometric contraction of the shoulder internal (subscapularis) and external rotators (infraspinatus, teres minor).

LONG-TERM

See chart on muscle flexibility (opposite).

The underlying cause of swimmer's shoulder needs to be determined to make sure the problem is not just an imbalance or impingement of the joint.

Failure to treat an instability allows the problem to worsen and presents the possibility of a rupture of tissue around the shoulder joint.

Tape the joint to help maintain the shoulder position and avoid closing down in the subacromial space.

Gradually build up strength around the shoulder as indicated in the strengthening program at the end of the chapter.

Swimmer's back

Swimmer's back—or spondylolisthesis—can develop as a result of stress fractures of the pars interarticularis of the lumbar spine.

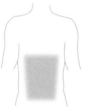

Swimmer's back: pain affects the lower back area.

Causes

Poor standing posture (sway posture), which leads to excessive movement into extension on one joint area, particularly the lumbar spine.

Repetitive stress as a result of turning at the end of the pool.

Strain as a result of poor head and body position in the water.

Repetitive hyperextension of the back, leading to stress on the vertebrae. Tends to occur while doing the butterfly as this movement can force contraction on the abdominals (pectoralis), which then leads to stress on the vertebral spine.

Injury can also occur during technique training; that is sudden movements and explosive action.

Signs and symptoms

Dull back ache, aggravated by activity.

Buttock pain.

Spasm in erector spinae muscles, indicated by tightness of the muscles on either side of the spine.

Hamstring spasm: limited raise of straight leg raise when tested.

Increased sway-back (lumbar lordosis) when standing.

Test for spondylolisthesis

Check to see whether your back aches when standing. Bend and rotate the trunk toward the opposite side of the spine.

Treatment

IMMEDIATE

Have a clear diagnosis of the problem by a qualified medical professional.

Reduce activity until pain recedes.

How to prevent

Correct your stroke technique.

Create a balanced training program: spend equal time on strokes.

Strengthen your deep stabilizer muscles (transversus abdominus) through the Pilates program at the end of this chapter.

Stretch and lengthen hamstrings. Follow the prescribed Pilates exercises at the end of this chapter.

Grade one/two spondylolisthesis slip: the joint has slipped in front of the other.

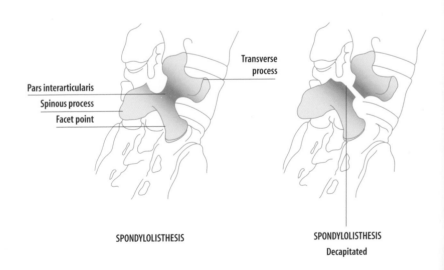

Transverse process

Pars interarticularis

Spinous process

Facet point

SPONDYLOLISTHESIS

SPONDYLOLISTHESIS
Decapitated

Swimmer's ankle

Swimmer's ankle is caused by repetitive kicking while swimming. If the ankle is not warmed up, or has an existing condition, the tendons at the top of the foot can become inflamed and tender.

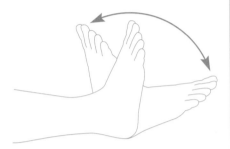

Make sure there is no limitation to the range of movement: point your toes to see whether or not you can achieve a straight foot without pain.

Causes

Tendonitis of the extensor tendons at the extensor retinaculum (thickened fibrous bands that hold the tendons down on the top of the foot) is caused by repeated extreme plantar flexion (foot pushing downward to point the toe) in flutter-and-dolphin kicking.

Signs and symptoms

The sound or feeling of bones clicking or rubbing against each other (crepitus) when the foot is passively pulled up toward the body.

Pain at the front of the ankle when the toe is pointed.

Treatment
IMMEDIATE

Apply ice to the top part of foot for ten minutes, or until the area is numb.

Reduce the amount of kicking action in the stroke when swimming.

Physiotherapy modalities.

Undertake soft tissue release to the front of the ankle.

Visit a physiotherapist for an ultrasound on the area of crepitus.

Stretch the muscles around the foot.

Rest by using pull-buoy while swimming.

LONG-TERM

May require joint mobilization to the ankle to help achieve this range.

Swimmer's elbow

Swimmer's elbow, or lateral epicondylitis, is an inflammation in the attachment of the extensor muscles of the elbow. It is usually caused through overuse during training, when there is repeated tugging at the muscle. If there is not adequate recovery time between periods of muscle activity (training), you may experience pain and inflammation on the outside of the elbow. Swimmer's elbow differs from tennis elbow because of its location (see diagram below).

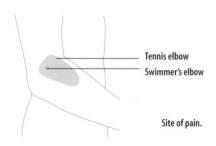

Tennis elbow
Swimmer's elbow

Site of pain.

Causes

Pain in the pull-through phase of the stroke (butterfly/breaststroke/free-style).

Dropping the elbow during the stroke (which may be because of a sore elbow). This pushes the body through the water less efficiently and places more strain on the extensor muscles of the elbow.

A change in style of swimming, or the stroke, can increase the risk of elbow pain and potential shoulder injuries.

Signs and symptoms

Pain and tenderness localized to the bony prominence at the outer "edge" of the elbow (lateral epicondyle).

Pain when gripping hands together to lift objects. This indicates weakness in the extensor and abductor of the hand at the wrist joint, known as the extensor carpi radialis brevis muscle.

Pain when conducting the Wrist Flexion test (see below).

Wrist Flexion test: elbow pain is reproduced if you force your wrist and hand into flexion while keeping the palm facing downward.

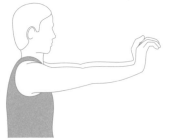

Treatment

IMMEDIATE

Place ice on the sore area for ten minutes (no longer) or until the area is numb.

Take anti-inflammatory tablets to reduce the inflammation.

Modify or avoid any painful activities for two weeks.

Enlist the services of a professional swimming coach to make sure your stroke is correct.

LONG-TERM

Have an assessment by a chartered physiotherapist.

Swimmer's knee

Within one year, one out of every three competitive swimmers will have an injury. Out of every three of these injuries, one will involve the knee.

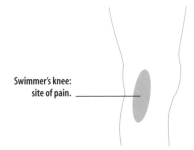

Swimmer's knee: site of pain.

Of all the injuries that occur in the knee, those affecting the kneecap are the most common. A variety of names have been given to this injury, most commonly chondromalacia or swimmer's knee.

Pain usually comes on gradually and

tends to be caused through the kicking action in breaststroke.

Unlike a skiing injury, where symptoms occur abruptly, the swimmer's knee pain occurs gradually over a period of weeks or even months. The pain is difficult to localize; however, it is usually around the kneecap.

Causes

Long-standing irritation of the medial collateral ligament.

Can be related to or irritated by incorrect twisting of the knee during breaststroke.

Signs and symptoms

Localized tenderness to the inside of the knee (medial collateral ligament).

Pain on valgus/external rotation.

Treatment

IMMEDIATE

Apply ice to the medial aspect of the knee for ten minutes, or until the area is numb.

Tape the knee to support it and prevent the ligament being pulled.

Visit a physiotherapist to receive ultrasound treatment to the ligament.

LONG-TERM

Correct your stroke technique.

Minimize breaststroke distance by cross-training with other strokes.

Correct the abnormal kicking action in the stroke.

Warm up adequately and correctly.

Increase your training distance gradually.

Breaststroke leg kick

Incorrect leg kick creates an abnormal strain on the kneecap and an incorrect gliding of the joint (patellofemoral) leading to problems.

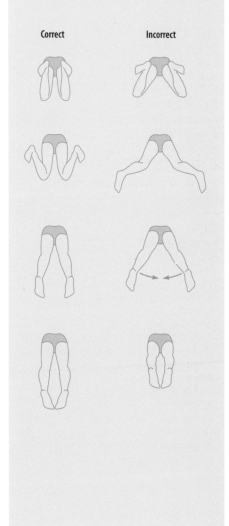

Correct   Incorrect

Pilates exercises to improve performance and prevent further injury

▌ Lengthen
▼ Balance
● Strengthen

	Swimmer's shoulder	Swimmer's back	Swimmer's ankle	Swimmer's elbow	Swimmer's knee
CORE EXERCISES					
curl up	●	●	●	●	●
diamond press	●			●	
floating arms	●			●	
four point challenge	▼	▼		▼	
hip opening			●		●
imprinting		●			
pelvic stability		●			●
neutral spine		●			
static standing balance		▼			▼
FOUNDATION EXERCISES					
arm circles	●			●	
arm opening				●	
dart	▌●			●	
hamstring lengthening		▌	▌		▌
long sitting stretch					●
mid back stretch	●			●	
neck rolls				●	
roll downs	●				
shoulder external rotation	●			●	
shoulder internal rotation	●			●	
shoulder push away	●			●	
shoulder rowing	●			●	
shoulder rotation	▌●				
side reach	●	▌●			
single knee kick		●	▌●		▌
spinal curls		●			●
standing squat			●		
star				●	
T-band balance			▼		▼

	Swimmer's shoulder	Swimmer's back	Swimmer's ankle	Swimmer's elbow	Swimmer's knee
threading the needle		●			
wall slides		▮	▮ ●		●
windows					
wrist openings				●	
PERFORMANCE PILATES					
bridging		●	●		●
double leg stretch	▮ ●	▮ ●	▮		▮
eccentric hamstrings					
heel drop			●		
hundred	●			●	●
leg pull prone	●	●		●	
lunge		●	●		●
mermaid	●				
oblique curl up		▮ ●			
open leg rocker		▮	▮		▮ ●
Pilates push up	▼ ●			●	
praying mantis	●	●		●	●
roll up					●
rolling like a ball		●	●		●
scissors		▮	▮		▮
shoulder challenge	●			●	
side kick series			●		●
single leg stretch		▮ ●	▮		●
sitting knee folds		▮			
superman	●	●		●	●
swimming	●		▮ ●		▮ ●
teaser		●	●		●
tennis ball raises			●		●
torpedo	●	●			●
wrist strengthening				●	

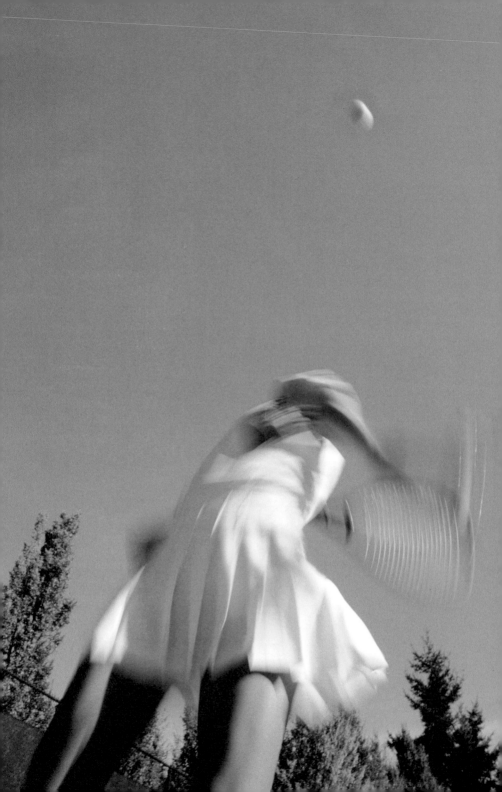

Tennis

Tennis requires agile movements, endurance, and strength, along with hand–eye and ball coordination skills. Each game involves controlled twisting in the upper body, so that the player can make successful strokes. Playing tennis regularly increases suppleness and tones the muscles. Common tennis injuries occur in the arms and legs. The upper limb problems are generally caused by how the ball is hit and by how the racket is held. Stress injuries in the lower limbs relate to the rapid changes of direction, sudden stopping and starting, and reaching for shots.

The Pilates exercises at the end of this chapter aim to improve your coordination through increased strength and muscle length in and around the upper body. With good core strength you can place your shoulder correctly to score a successful shot. This control can prevent injury problems as well as improve your game.

Common tennis injuries

Tennis elbow

Lateral epicondylitis, commonly known as tennis elbow, is an inflammatory problem that causes pain and tenderness on the outside of the elbow. It is an overuse injury and damage occurs when there is repeated tugging of the extensor muscle, where it is attached to the elbow.

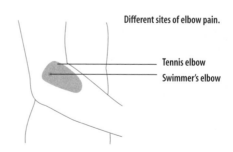

Different sites of elbow pain.

Tennis elbow
Swimmer's elbow

Causes

A poor stroke technique, particularly on the backhand. The wrist needs to remain straight and firm and not bend during the backhand stroke. Bending often happens because the forearm muscles are not strong enough to withstand the ball's impact on the racket.

Too-tight racket strings that bring about stress in the arm.

145

Playing with heavy-duty balls or with wet balls.

Signs and symptoms

Pain and tenderness is felt in the elbow area.

Pain is also felt in the gripping hand, or when lifting objects. This indicates a weakness to the extensor carpi radialis brevis muscle (see page 163).

Treatment

IMMEDIATE

Place an ice pack on the tender area for ten minutes or until the area is numb.

Take anti-inflammatory tablets to reduce inflammation.

Take a break from tennis for two weeks, or modify your stroke.

Ask a tennis coach to look at your racket and playing technique particularly when you play a backhand.

LONG-TERM

Have an assessment with a chartered physiotherapist who will look at your cervical spine and check for any movement restriction of your neural

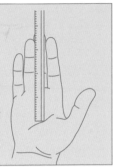

Measuring your ideal grip size

The ideal racket grip circumference should equal, or be larger than, the distance from the middle of your palm (check the line is level with the middle finger and base of your thumb) to the tip of your ring finger.

tissue that may be referring pain to the elbow area.

You need to modify your playing technique to prevent tennis elbow so take note of the following:

Risk factors for tennis elbow:

1. Age of player. From 30 years of age upward the muscles may not respond as well to stresses.

2. Incorrect grip size, which can lead to an over-tight grip.

3. Using a metal racket, which creates vibration from the racket into the arm.

4. Tiredness, as a result of playing more than two hours a day.

5. Incorrect backhand technique, creating excessive motion of the elbow joint and/or arm muscles.

How to prevent

Do some forearm stretching.

Have an adequate warm-up session before your game.

Gradually build up the speed and power of strokes before starting your game.

Only practice your forehand during your warm-up. Or if your elbow is tender, work on correcting your technique.

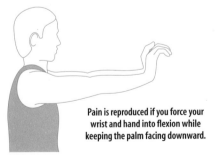

Pain is reproduced if you force your wrist and hand into flexion while keeping the palm facing downward.

Gradually build up the time you spend playing.

Rotator cuff pain

Causes

The shoulder rotator cuff muscles and tendons can become strained from the backward movement of the serve or during overhead actions.

Rotator cuff area

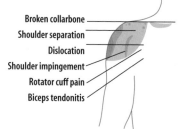

Broken collarbone
Shoulder separation
Dislocation
Shoulder impingement
Rotator cuff pain
Biceps tendonitis

Signs and symptoms

A pain is felt at the front of the shoulder joint as the hand is placed behind the back to serve.

There is pain at the back of the shoulder joint perhaps because the shoulder joints sliding backward and forward in the joint space (a subluxing joint).

Muscle weakness around the shoulder blade. This can be indicated by the shoulder blade sticking out when the hand is placed behind the back.

Weakness to the external rotators of the shoulder, indicated by a limited ability to turn the upper arm outward as compared to inward. Check for discomfort by placing your hand behind your head. Compare this to putting the back of your hand on your lower back.

Treatment

IMMEDIATE

P.R.I.C.E.

Take anti-inflammatory tablets to reduce inflammation.

If painful, take a rest from tennis for two weeks, or keep serves low and under shoulder height.

Have some physiotherapy to help improve local joint mobilization.

Practice tightening the rotator cuff muscles with your arm by your side but without moving the shoulder muscles.

LONG-TERM

Keep modifying your serve. This will help prevent aggravation of the inflammation and pulling too much on the rotator cuff tendons and muscles.

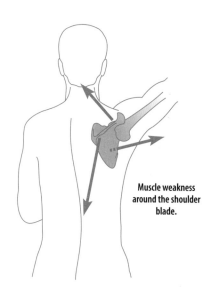

Muscle weakness around the shoulder blade.

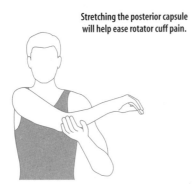

Stretching the posterior capsule will help ease rotator cuff pain.

1. Improve shoulder internal rotation. (subscapularis, teres major) (see page 163).

2. Stretch posterior capsule (see diagram, above).

3. Build up the shoulder muscles by doing Pilates push-up, diamond press, and shoulder push away (see pages 217, 170 and 191).

How to prevent

Check your range of movement in the muscle around the shoulder joint to determine whether there are any muscle imbalances around the joint.

Respect the pain you are experiencing. Limit the amount of tennis you play until the pain is absent.

Get a professional to check your overhead stroke techniques.

Check that the strings of your racket are not too tight.

Rotator Cuff Movements tests

Test to indicate balance of rotation around the shoulder. You need to have a range of rotation in the shoulder that is 180 degrees or greater when the arm is held in a 90 degree or abducted position.

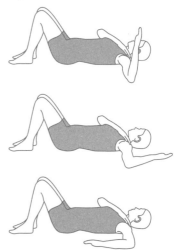

Biceps tendonitis

This is a condition where swelling and pain occurs at the biceps tendon at the front of the shoulder joint.

Causes

This is an overuse injury, caused by putting excessive pressure on the biceps muscle when serving and playing overhead shots.

Signs and symptoms

A localized tenderness in the biceps tendon at the front of the shoulder joint.

Shoulder is painful when moved forward and upward.

Pain when shoulder is turned inward.

Treatment

IMMEDIATE

Modify the strokes that aggravate the pain. If still painful after a week stop playing to allow recovery.

Place an ice pack on the inflamed area for ten minutes, or until the area is numb.

Take anti-inflammatory tablets to reduce localized swelling and pain.

Have physiotherapy, plus localized ultrasound treatment to reduce pain and swelling.

Passive stretching of the tendon using PNF (proprioceptive neuromuscular facilitation) techniques. These balancing techniques help to improve your strength and stamina.

How to prevent

See Rotator cuff pain, pages 147–148.

Muscle imbalance

The rotator cuff muscles around the shoulder are responsible for the stability of the shoulder joint in its capsule during upper-limb movements. The rotator cuff muscles work as couples, so if the shoulder is turned inward the muscles that turn the shoulder out will lengthen. This is called forced couples. Problems around the shoulder occur when the forced couples are not working properly creating a muscle imbalance.

The four muscles of the rotator cuff muscle group—supraspinatus, infraspinatus, subscapularis, and teres minor—maintain the joint in a stable position when the shoulder moves.

Causes

Tightness of the internal rotators (subscapularis) and weakness of the external rotators (teres minor and infra-spinatus). These restrictions are noticeable at the end of a serve as a slowing-down movement.

Weakness of the scapular stabilizer muscle (lower trapezius and/or serratus anterior). Tightness is felt in the pectoralis major/minor and anterior deltoid muscles. This can lead to rounded shoulders and/or a reduction in the ability to open your arms and reach up for a serve.

Tightness of the latissimus dorsi muscle, which reduces the ability to do a full stroke.

Loss of full forward flexion and abduction—where the arm moves out from the side, and there is external rotation of the shoulder. Tightness will also influence the thoracic and lumbar spine by increasing the curves in this area.

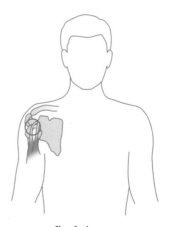

Site of pain.

The difference between biceps tendonitis and a biceps rupture

Tendonitis is gradual onset of pain in the area.
A rupture is a sudden, sharp tearing pain in the front of the elbow joint or lower front upper arm.
A rupture shows visibly when you bend your elbow.
You may also be able to feel the gap in the muscle.

Signs and symptoms

Loss of range in motion in actions such as serving.

Inability to attain a long-reach action during serving.

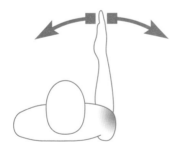

Positive impingement tests.

Treatment

IMMEDIATE

Application of P.R.I.C.E. techniques.

Take anti-inflammatory tablets.

Modify serves, keeping them low and under shoulder height. If still painful after a week stop playing to allow recovery.

Have physiotherapy to aid joint mobilization within a pain-free range.

Practice tightening rotator cuff muscles with arms by your side but without moving the shoulder muscles.

LONG-TERM

Modify your serve. This will help prevent aggravating the inflammation and pulling too much on the rotator cuff tendons and muscles.

1. Improve shoulder internal rotation. (subscapularis, teres major).

2. Build up your shoulder muscles by doing Pilates push up (page 217), diamond press (page 170), and shoulder push away (page 191).

How to prevent

Do some forearm stretching.

Have an adequate warm-up session.

Gradually build up the speed and power of strokes before starting your game.

Gradually build up the time you play during a session.

Undertake shoulder program (see pages 189–193) regularly.

Back strain

Back problems occur in tennis because of attempts to play shots while the back is in a vulnerable position such as bending, stretching, or turning in to a laterally flexed position (serving). Muscle strain can also happen because of rapid movements of the upper body.

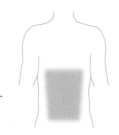

Area of back strain.

Causes

Performing a back twist while serving.

Poor muscle control when trying to complete a shot.

Over-reaching at the end of shots because of poor muscle control to slow movements down.

Signs and symptoms

Nonspecific back pain.

Aches in the middle of the back.

Treatment

IMMEDIATE

Take anti-inflammatory tablets to reduce pain and inflammation.

Improve the contraction of the supporting muscles of the back.

Undertake core exercise program (see pages 169-178).

LONG-TERM

Your way of playing may need modifying for long-term relief:

1 Have some coaching to improve your stroke technique.

2 Undertake a comprehensive abdominal program to give your back more support (see pages 169-178).

Tennis leg (torn calf muscle)

Tennis leg is when a sudden, acute pain is felt in the calf (gastrocnemius muscle). Most commonly, fibers of the muscle tear when the player rushes for a shot.

Causes

Failure to do warm-up stretches before a game.

Repeated rushing for the net which involves slapping the foot down while the knee is extended.

An extreme lunge forward.

Sudden slowing down from a run without the muscle being warmed up properly first.

Signs and symptoms

A sudden pain in the calf, which feels as though someone has hit you in the calf with a racket or ball. The pain is so intense you have to stop playing. The muscles can take four to six weeks to heal.

Treatment

IMMEDIATE

Apply P.R.I.C.E. techniques.

Do regular circular movements of the

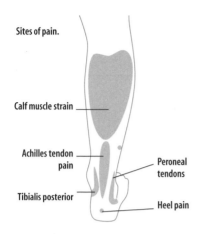

Sites of pain.

Calf muscle strain

Achilles tendon pain

Peroneal tendons

Tibialis posterior

Heel pain

Achilles tendonitis

The Achilles tendon, the largest tendon in the body, connects the gastrocnemius and soleus muscles to the heel, transferring the force of their contractions to lift the heel. There are two types of Achilles tendonitis. One, an inflammatory condition that occurs because of overuse, the other, a degeneration of the tendons.

Causes

Turning the foot over while running.

Straining Achilles tendon while jumping.

Many years spent jumping or running.

Playing tennis without firstly getting fit.

Playing on a different surface.

A change in footwear.

Calf weakness.

Restriction when lifting foot upward.

Excessive pronation of the ankle and foot, causing the Achilles tendon to pull off-center and become inflamed.

Signs and symptoms

Severe tendon pain that can be widespread.

Tight gastrocnemius muscle.

Burning type pain around the tendon.

Involves the entire thickness of the tendon.

Gradual onset of tendon pain.

Pain and/or stiffness in tendon first thing in the morning.

Tenderness that is uncomfortable to touch. Often a deep, marked swelling that moves with the tendon.

foot while your leg is elevated. Doctor may advise to keep your leg in a raised position, so that it is higher than the heart, for 48 hours.

Take anti-inflammatory tablets to reduce pain and inflammation.

Use a heel raise in your shoe if you are unable to walk on the flat without sharp pain.

Maintain range-of-motion exercises in the early stages of injury. Do not stretch as this may lead to more fibers being pulled.

LONG-TERM

Rest while the muscle heals.

Take medical advice for when you should start playing again.

How to prevent

Do warm-up stretching exercises before each game.

Undertake a sufficient lengthening program for the calf muscles.

How to prevent tennis injuries

FITNESS EVALUATION

Always play to your level of fitness—choose competitors of a similar level or only slightly better.

TRAINING TECHNIQUES

1. Have some coaching lessons to review your forehand and backhand techniques.

2. Improve your overall fitness to play tennis, for example work out in the gym or go running.

3. Play tennis to a skill level and with a frequency and intensity that does not produce an overuse injury.

EQUIPMENT

Shoes

Buy well-fitting shoes that can cope with extreme movements, such as stop/start bursts. Check that the design accommodates side as well as forward and backward motions. The outer sole needs to adapt well to playing surfaces. The middle of the sole should absorb impact forces well.

Racket

1. Choose a racket to suit your skill level. Check tightness of strings for injury prevention.

2. Oversized rackets are best as they have large "sweet spots" that reduce the number of off-center hits, and lessen vibration and shock load on the arm. They allow slow-swing players to enjoy the game.

A COMPARISON OF PLAYING SURFACES

Consistent, unforgiving surface	Consistent, forgiving surface
Hard surface—asphalt/concrete	Softer surface—clay
Has no shock absorbency.	Slow play and slippery surface.
Limited ability to slide to the ball. With a fast ball need better footwork and earlier preparation.	Pace of ball is slower.
Need speedy reactions. The fast pace of the ball increases the impact force on the upper limbs and creates other problems.	More time to reach the ball and prepare the racket to hit it.
	Lower occurrence of knee and foot problems.

Treatment

IMMEDIATE

Stop playing while the tendon is tender. If you experience any pain as you raise up on your toes, the condition can easily become chronic.

Take anti-inflammatory tablets.

Doing gentle heel raises can help resolve acute condition in three to four weeks.

LONG-TERM

Try to reduce jumping when playing.

Carry on following "immediate" treatments until pain settles.

Undertake a muscle strengthening program to lengthen the ankle muscles under tension (see heel drops page 207).

How to prevent

Stretch out the calf and hamstring muscles that pull the foot upward.

Practice tensing your lower leg to lengthen the Achilles tendons.

Ankle inversion injury

Ankle sprains are by far the most common injury in sports, including tennis. Injury results from the ankle rolling over, straining the peroneus longus and tibialis posterior muscle. A sprain will also happen if the foot is forced upward as the ankle twists.

Causes

Bad landing from a jump.

Stepping or landing on an opponent's foot.

Suddenly changing direction.

Abrupt slowing down during a run.

Playing on an uneven surface.

Weak peroneal muscles (on the outside of the ankle).

A tight Achilles tendon.

A previous ankle injury.

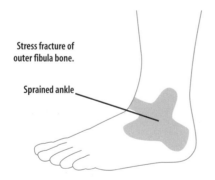

Stress fracture of outer fibula bone.

Sprained ankle

Signs and symptoms

Experiencing a popping or tearing sensation and pain in the ankle.

Pain when the ankle is touched and at rest.

Being unable to walk on the ankle without pain.

Swelling and bruising on the side of the foot.

Treatment

IMMEDIATE

Application of P.R.I.C.E. techniques.

Take anti-inflammatory tablets to reduce pain and tenderness.

Try to write the alphabet in the air with your foot without experiencing pain.

LONG-TERM

Achieve a good sense of balance in the ankle by building up its strength.

Practise balance exercises.

Limit the amount you play until you are pain-free.

Try not to rely on an ankle support as the ankle will stay weak and more prone to injury.

How to prevent

Try to maintain good strength and coordination around the ankle joint by undertaking the Pilates exercises at the end of this chapter.

Plantar fasciitis

Pain is felt under the sole of the foot at the anterior margin of the heel bone (the calcaneum). The pain is caused by overuse and by irritation and inflammation to the bands of the fascia—the tight, thickened bands of fibers along the sole of the foot.

Causes

Overstretching of the plantar muscles as a result of poor foot posture.

Standing for too long or excessive running.

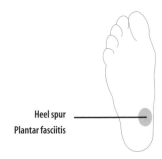

Heel spur
Plantar fasciitis

Wearing tennis shoes with inadequate arch support.

Having flexible arches of the feet.

Having a tight Achilles tendon.

Signs and symptoms

One-sided pain on the sole of the foot.

Pain in the foot when stepping out of bed.

Pain aggravated when playing tennis.

Treatment

IMMEDIATE

Put icepack on the tender area for ten minutes or until the area is numb.

Take anti-inflammatory tablets.

Use a heel raise in the shoe.

LONG-TERM

1. Keep your feet flat on the floor and attempt to separate all your toes—either as a group or individually.

2. Pull your toes back, so that the pads stay on the floor but the knuckles of the toe joints raise up.

3. Use a heel pad.

4. Get advice on buying correct, supportive tennis shoes.

How to prevent

Increase your general flexibility of legs by starting a lengthening program for the hamstring and quadriceps muscles (see pages 208-215).

Pilates exercises to improve performance and prevent further injury

▼ Balance
● Strength
▌ Lengthen

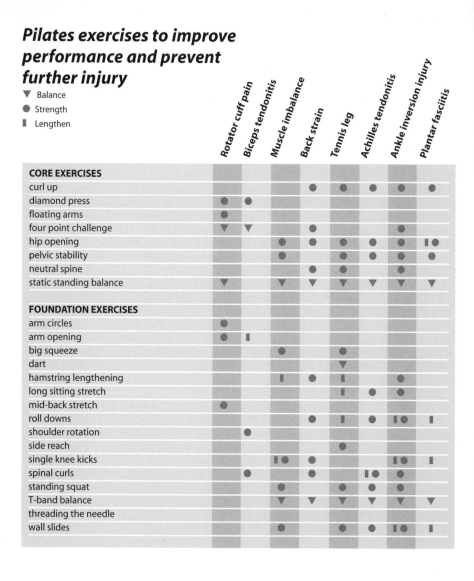

	Rotator cuff pain	Biceps tendonitis	Muscle imbalance	Back strain	Tennis leg	Achilles tendonitis	Ankle inversion injury	Plantar fasciitis
CORE EXERCISES								
curl up				●	●	●	●	●
diamond press	●	●						
floating arms	●							
four point challenge	▼	▼		●			●	
hip opening			●	●	●	●	●	▌●
pelvic stability			●		●	●	●	●
neutral spine				●	●		●	
static standing balance	▼		▼	▼	▼	▼	▼	▼
FOUNDATION EXERCISES								
arm circles	●							
arm opening	●	▌						
big squeeze			●		●			
dart					▼			
hamstring lengthening			▌	●	▌		●	
long sitting stretch					▌	●	●	
mid-back stretch	●							
roll downs				●	▌	●	▌●	▌
shoulder rotation		●						
side reach					●			
single knee kicks			▌●	●			▌●	▌
spinal curls		●		●		▌●	●	
standing squat			●		●	●	●	
T-band balance			▼	▼	▼	▼	▼	▼
threading the needle								
wall slides			●		●	●	▌●	▌

	Rotator cuff pain	Biceps tendonitis	Muscle imbalance	Back strain	Tennis leg	Achilles tendonitis	Ankle inversion injury	Plantar fasciitis
PERFORMANCE PILATES								
bridging					●	●	●	●
double leg stretch			●	●	●			
eccentric hamstrings			●		●			
hundred	●	●	●		●	●		
knee/leg circles					I		I	
lean forward bending			●		●		●	
leg pull prone		●			I			
lunge		●			●		●	
open leg rocker			●	●	●			
Pilates push up		●						
praying mantis		●					●	
roll up			●		I			
rolling like a ball						I		
scissors			●	●	●	I		I
shoulder challenge								
side kick series			●		●		●	
side rolls					I			
single leg stretch			●	●	●	●	●	
superman		●						
swimming	●	●	●	●	●	●		I
teaser		●			●			
tennis ball raises			●		I ●	●	●	●
torpedo					●	●		
waist twists in standing	●							

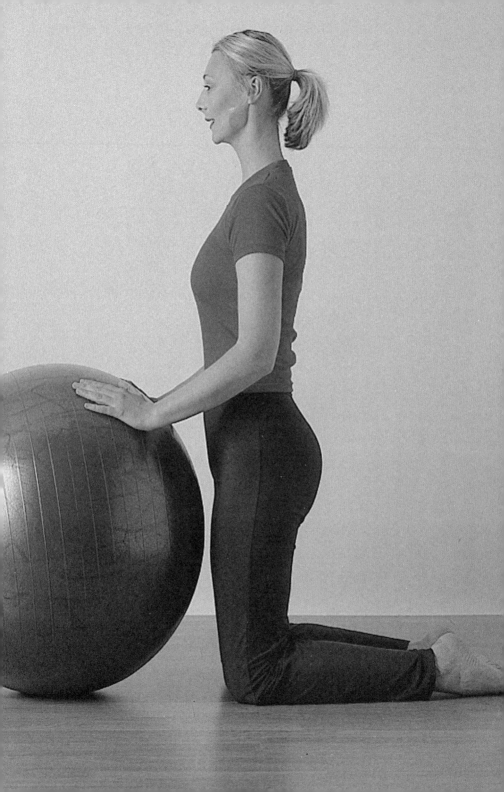

Principles of Pilates

Before you begin your exercise program, it is very important to understand the various aspects of Pilates. This will help you to make the most of your Pilates program and allow you to achieve your goal of rehabilitation and prevention of further injury.

Relaxation

Relaxing regulates your breathing, slows your pulse, and helps to relieve stress. It is important to remain relaxed while performing the Pilates movements to avoid straining or pulling any muscles. Being relaxed will also help you achieve the movement easier.

Concentration

1. Focus

The ability to focus on the muscles as you practice Pilates will help you to perform movement correctly. Pilates exercises need a constant level of awareness.

2. Proprioception

Proprioception is the awareness of the correct sequence for each exercise. It is actually a balanced state between movement and the movement pattern.

3. Correct movement patterns

The correct movement pattern is a balance between three systems: passive elements (muscles that do not contract), active elements (muscles that contract and relax), and the neutral or control system (coordinates the movement).

Alignment

Correct alignment is required when the body is in motion. Bad patterns of behavior may affect your posture and muscle balance and lead to aches and pains. Pilates rebalances your muscles for better body alignment and improves your posture and your resistance to injury.

Breathing

Breathing correctly when exercising can be the difference between straining to complete an exercise and performing the move easily. Correct breathing involves tightening the abdominal muscles. By controlling the abdominal muscles when doing Pilates, you create a strong core from which all movements originate.

Breathing method

Before commencing the movement breathe in to prepare. Breathe wide and full into your back. As you begin the movement, breathe out and contract your lower abdominals. Breathe in as you return to neutral position or before commencing the next stage.

Centering

All too often we neglect our core muscles: the neck, shoulder blades, trunk, and pelvis (see opposite). These muscles form the center of our body, or, as Joseph Pilates coined them, our "powerhouse." Coordination between the core areas enables us to establish good, safe movement patterns.

Finding your core

Neck

Position: Keep the length in the back of the neck, jaw relaxed.

Muscles used: Deep neck flexors.

Shoulders and shoulder blades

Position: Keep the shoulder blades drawn down the back.

Muscles used: lower trapezius, serratus anterior.

Trunk

Position: Engage the lower stomach muscles.

Muscles: transversus abdominis, multifidis.

Pelvis

Position: Keep the tail bone down, maintaining neutral spine position (see page 177).

Muscles used: transversus abdominis, balance with gluteals, hip abductors, adductors.

Coordination and flowing movements

When you have practiced Pilates for a few weeks, you will undoubtedly notice an improvement in your overall coordination, as well as a more "flowing" aspect to your movements.

As Pilates movements are not isolated (because the body does not move this way), it is easier to achieve a sense of flow and coordination from head to toe. In sports, a sudden, jerky, or unexpected movement can cause injury. Integrating Pilates in to your exercise program will help to eliminate these potential injuries (see calf strain page 36 and hamstring strain page 46).

Lengthening

The lengthening movements achieved in Pilates will help you stretch the muscle to its full range, to work both the lengthening and supporting muscle and establish correct muscle balance.

Sequencing

The sequence in which you perform each Pilates exercise is important to enable you to achieve good quality of movement. As Pilates is a progressive form of movement (each move should seamlessly flow into the next one), it is important to follow the steps for each exercise in their specified order. Following the correct sequence for a movement will help you to avoid injury and create a balanced state for your posture. Any imbalance can be caused by repetitive

traversus abdominis

1. Draw up the pelvic floor, imagining the area at the base of your pelvis moving up along the front of your spine out toward the top of your head.

2. Move in the widest possible arc, visualizing a string pulled upwardly from the pelvic floor through the top of your head.

3. Draw the navel in and up, as if to tighten an airline seat across the base of the pelvis.

4. Move your head forward until your gaze is horizontal with the floor.

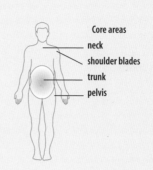

Core areas
neck
shoulder blades
trunk
pelvis

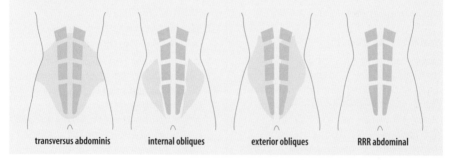

| transversus abdominis | internal obliques | exterior obliques | RRR abdominal |

incorrect movements, or incorrect posture in the static position (page 178).

Once you have mastered a move, it is possible to move onto the progressive exercise. For example, the diamond press exercise (page 170), lays down the foundation for the dart (page 183) and shoulder rotation exercises (pages 189-190).

Once these movements are practiced correctly it is then possible to move onto the performance exercises for this area, such as swimming (page 228).

Beginning your program

Begin with the core exercises (page 169). These will help to teach you how to find your "powerhouse" and establish a firm foundation from which to advance.

Foundation exercises build on this beginning, concentrating on lengthening and strengthening the muscles.

Performance exercises are slightly more advanced and should be attempted only after gaining complete confidence and competency at the previous two levels.

Note: Always follow the specific exercise sequence to prevent injury or imbalance.

Muscle imbalance

When an injury occurs your muscles can overcompensate and create a muscle imbalance. Muscles can be defined into two groups: mobilizers and stabilizers.

Mobilizers

Mobilizers are found close to the body's surface and tend to cross two joints. They are made up of fast twitch fibers that produce power but lack endurance: the muscle contraction builds up tension in the muscle fibers rapidly, but they quickly become tired. With time and use muscles can become tightened and shortened.

Stabilizer muscles

Stabilizers are located deep down, near to the skeleton. They tend to cross one joint and are made up of slow twitch muscle fibers, which help with endurance. This group of muscles helps to maintain posture and works against gravity. With time, the muscles become weak and long.

Causes of muscle imbalance

Injury to the area, leading to an inflammation in the tissue.

Pain or restriction in movement.

Poor technique during the activity.

Incorrect recruitment of the muscle (poor motor control).

Poor posture during the activity.

Rehabilitation of muscle imbalance

Before undertaking any exercise, it is important to assess any evidence of muscle imbalance.

Assessing muscle imbalance

1. Complete the following movements as shown on pages 164–165.

   Swimming

   Hip abduction

   Curl up

   Neutral spine

   Pilates push-up

   Floating arms

   Does your posture remain stable during these exercises? Do you need to use other parts of your body in order to achieve the movement?

2. Identify the strength and function of individual muscles.

3. Determine the flexibility of the muscles needed in your sport. Lack of flexibility in muscles and muscle groups may hamper your ability to undertake particular movements. Once you have identified where you need flexibility, any tightness can then be corrected.

Methods to correct muscle-length limitation

Palpation of specific muscles

Taping the areas.

Following the recommended Pilates program on page 166–167.

Mobilizer muscles
Local superficial muscles

Iliopsoas

Hamstrings

Rectus femoris

Tensor fasciae latae
hip adductors

Piriformis

Rectus abdominis

External obliques

Quadratus lumborum

Erector spinae,
Sternocleidomastoid

Upper trapezius

Levator scapulae

Rhomboids

Pectoralis major / minor

Scalenes

Stabilizer muscles
Local deep muscles

Transversus abdominis

Internal obliques

Gluteus medius

Vastus medialis oblique

Serratus anterior

Lower trapezius

Deep neck flexors

Global intermediate depth

Gluteus maximus

Quadriceps

Iliopsoas

Subscapularis
infraspinatus

Upper trapezius

Quadratus lumborum

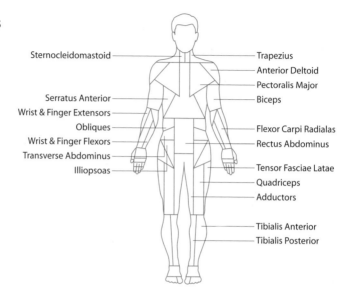

Sternocleidomastoid — Trapezius

— Anterior Deltoid

— Pectoralis Major

Serratus Anterior — Biceps

Wrist & Finger Extensors

Obliques — Flexor Carpi Radialas

Wrist & Finger Flexors — Rectus Abdominus

Transverse Abdominus

Illiopsoas — Tensor Fasciae Latae

— Quadriceps

— Adductors

— Tibialis Anterior

— Tibialis Posterior

Sternocleidomastoid — Trapezius

Mid Trapezius — Posterior Deltoid

Infraspinatus — Teres Major

Latissimus Dorsi — Biceps

— Extensor Muscles

Quadratus Lumborum — Wrist & Finger Extensors

Gluteus Maximus

Gluteus Medius

Gluteus Minimus — Tensor Fasciae Latae

— Biceps Femoris

— Semimembranosus

Gastronemius — Gastronemius

— Soleus (deep)

Swimming (see page 228)

Method: Lie face down on the floor, with your arms and legs extended, shoulder-width apart. Lift your left leg and right arm up and away from you. Stretch your fingers and toes out. Release and allow your arms and legs to return slowly to the floor.

Incorrect movement pattern: gluteals tighten before the hamstrings; the back twists and both sides of the back tighten; the leg twists as it is raised and has limited flexibility.

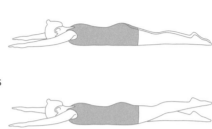

Hip opening (see page 174)

Method: Lie on your side, knees bent, your lower arm out below your head, so that it is in line with your body. Engage your lower stomach muscles and slowly open your top leg, moving it away from the bottom one, keeping your feet together. Hold and lower.

Incorrect movement pattern: hip moves upward; leg and body twist.

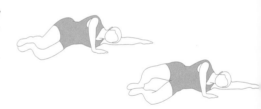

Curl up (see page 169)

Method: Lie on your back, knees bent and feet hip-width apart, hands behind your head. Engage your lower stomach muscles, then gently release the muscles at the back of your neck and allow your chin to fold on to your chest. Breathe out, then slowly curl your trunk up toward your knees. Curl up to the hold point (see diagram). Keep your lower stomach muscles engaged and slowly uncurl down.

Incorrect movement pattern: neck pain; allowing the pelvis to move.

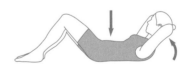

Neutral spine (see page 177)

Method: Lie on the floor, with your knees bent, feet hip-width apart, shoulder blades slightly lengthened down your back. You forehead should be parallel to the ceiling and your jaw relaxed. Gently and without discomfort, tilt your pelvis forward and backward. The middle area of this movement is the neutral position for your pelvis.

Incorrect movement pattern: neck pain; allowing the pelvis to move.

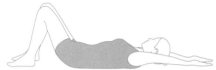

Pilates push-up (see page 217)

Method: Stand with your shoulders relaxed, feet hip-width apart. Roll down until your hands reach the floor (bend your knees if necessary). When your hands reach the floor, walk your hands forwards until your hands are aligned with your shoulders. Your body should be in a straight line. Bend your elbows and allow your body to move down to the floor. Hold, and push your chest away from the floor. Return to standing.

Incorrect movement pattern: arched back; shoulders move upward; wrist pain; chin pokes out; shoulder blades "pop out."

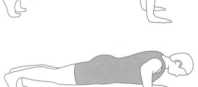

Floating arms (see page 172)

Method: Stand with your feet hip-width apart, knees slightly bent, arms hanging loosely by your sides. Rest your right hand on your left shoulder. Engage your lower stomach muscles, then allow your left arm to float up. When you feel your left shoulder lift under your hand, allow your arm to lower to the starting position.

Incorrect movement pattern: using your neck muscles; ribs move; whole body shifts as the arm raises.

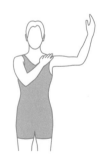

Pilates exercises to improve movement

❙ Lengthen
▼ Balance
● Strength

	Swimming	Hip opening	Curl up	Neutral spine	Pilates push up	Floating arms
CORE EXERCISES						
curl up		●	●			
diamond press					●	●
floating arms					●	●
four point challenge	●		●			
pelvic stability	●	●	●			
neutral spine		●	●			
static standing balance		●				
FOUNDATION EXERCISES						
arm circles					●	●
big squeeze	●					
breathing patterns			●		●	●
dart	●				●	●
hamstring lengthening	●					
long sitting stretch		●				
neck rolls	●					
shoulder external rotation					●	●
shoulder push away					●	●
shoulder rowing					●	●
shoulder external rotation					●	●
shoulder internal rotation					●	●
side reach		●				
single knee kicks	●					
spinal curls		●				
standing squat	●					

	Swimming	Hip opening	Curl up	Neutral spine	Pilates push up	Floating arms
star					●	●
T-band balance		●				
threading the needle						
wall slides	●	●				
PERFORMANCE PILATES						
bridging	●					
double leg stretch					●	●
hundred					●	●
knee/leg circles	●	●				
lunge	●	●				
obliques		●				
open leg rocker		●				
Pilates push up					●	●
praying mantis					●	●
roll up					●	●
scissors	●					
side kick series		●				
side rolls		●				
single leg stretch		●				
sitting knee folds		●				
superman					●	●
swimming	●				●	●
teaser					●	●
torpedo		●				

The Exercises

Core exercises

curl up

diamond press

floating arms

four point challenge

hip opening

pelvic stability

imprinting

neutral spine

static standing balance

Foundation exercises

arm circles

arm opening

big squeeze

breathing patterns

dart

hamstring lengthening

long sitting stretch

mid-back stretch

neck rolls

roll downs

shoulder external rotation

shoulder internal rotation

shoulder push away

shoulder rotation control

shoulder rowing

side reach

single knee kicks

spinal curls

standing squat

star

T-band balance

threading the needle

wall slides

windows

wrist openings

Performance exercises

bridging

double leg stretch

eccentric hamstrings

heel drop

hundred

knee /leg circles

lean forward bending

leg pull back

leg pull prone

lunge

mermaid

oblique curl ups

open leg rocker

Pilates push-up

praying mantis

roll ups

rolling like a ball

scissors

shoulder challenge

side kick series

side rolls

single leg stretch

sitting knee folds

superman

swimming

teaser

tennis ball raises

torpedo

waist twists in standing

wrist strengthening

Curl up (abdominal curl)

SPORTS: ALL

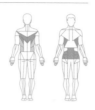

Focus
To strengthen abdominals
To establish correct sequence for abdominal curl
To enhance body alignment
To strengthen trunk stability

Breathe OUT as you curl up. Breathe IN as you lower.

Method

Muscles
Lengthen
Quadratus lumborum
Latissimus dorsi

1. Lie on your back, knees bent, and feet hip-width apart. Rest your hands behind your head, keeping your elbows wide. Your pelvis should be in the neutral position.

Strengthen
Rectus abdominus
Transversus abdominus
Obliques
Deep neck flexors
Scapular stabilizers
Serratus anterior
Lower trapezius

2. Engage your lower stomach muscles to create a strong core. Gently release the muscles at the back of your neck and allow your chin to fold on to your chest. Imagine that you are holding a small peach under your chin—be careful not to squash it or let it go.

3. Soften your chest bone and feel your ribs widen on the in-breath.

4. Breathe out, then slowly curl your trunk up toward your knees. Keep your pelvis still, ensuring that you are using your stomach muscles to perform the movement, not your hips.

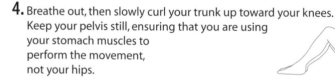

5. Curl up to the hold point (see diagram).

GOOD FOR:

Low-back pain
Rotator cuff pain
Biceps tendonitis
Patellofemoral pain
Achilles tendonitis
Hamstring strain
Tronchanteric hip pain

6. Keeping your lower stomach muscles engaged, slowly uncurl back to the starting position.

Common mistakes to avoid
Be careful not to pull yourself in to position through your hips.

Don't lose your neutral pelvis position.

Don't drop your chin too far forward. Keep a long, elegant sensation in the neck.

Diamond press

SPORTS: BASEBALL, BASKETBALL, CYCLING, FOOTBALL, GOLF, HOCKEY, SAILING, SOCCER, SWIMMING, TENNIS, WINDSURFING

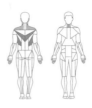

Focus

To develop awareness of the shoulder blades
To enhance the activation of the stabilizing muscle for the shoulder blade
To work the deep neck flexors
To encourage a feeling of length in the spine

Breathe OUT at starting position and to engage the abdominal muscle. Breathe IN when raising your upper body.

Muscles

Lengthen

Upper trapezius
Levator scapulae
Neck extensors

Strengthen

Lower trapezius
Serratus anterior
Latissimus dorsi
Rhomboids infraspinatus
Teres minor
Lower abdominals

Method

1. Lie on your front with your feet parallel and hip-width apart. Create a diamond shape with your arms by placing your fingertips together just above your forehead. Your elbows should be open and your shoulder blades relaxed.

2. Take a deep breath in. Then, engage your lower stomach muscle, while breathing out.

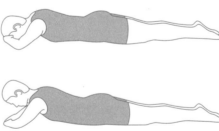

3. Breathe in and lengthen through your spine. Breathe out and pull your abdominal muscles in and pull the shoulder blades down and back toward your waist.

4. Gently tuck in your chin to lengthen the back of your neck and lift your head one or two inches off the floor. Looking down at the floor, imagine a cord pulling you from the top of your head. Notice the connection down into the small of your back. Don't push on your elbows. Think about them connecting with your waist. Keep your lower stomach lifted and your ribs on the floor.

5. Breathe out, keeping your stomach pulled in, then slowly lower down to the floor.

Variation

To advance this move further, repeat the above steps. When your head and upper body are raised, slowly slide your hands away from your body, along the floor, making sure your shoulder blades are down. Turn your hand palms inward, so that your little fingers are closest to the ground. Take the movement further upward by lifting your chest until your feel a tightness in your back and under the arms. Slowly lower and return to the starting position.

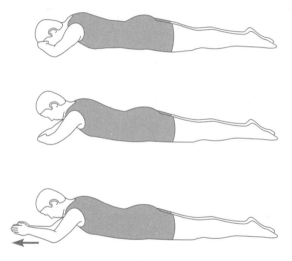

Common mistakes to avoid

Be careful not to raise your head and look upward as this can put strain on the back of your neck.

Make sure that your abdominals are pulled in tight at all times.

Don't force your shoulder blades—the sensation should be of stretching, rather than forcing.

GOOD FOR:

Rotator cuff pain
Swimmer's shoulder
Biceps tendonitis
Acromioclavicular joint sprain

Floating arms

SPORTS: BASEBALL, CYCLING, GOLF, SAILING, SKIING, SWIMMING, TENNIS, WINDSURFING

Focus

To enhance the correct movement of the shoulder (humerus)
in relation to the scapular movement

To create a differential movement of the arm to shoulder blade

To stabilize the shoulder muscles (lower trapezius, serratus anterior)

To reduce tension in the neck

Breathe OUT as you raise your arm.
Breathe IN as you lower your arm.

Method

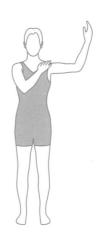

1. Stand up straight with your feet hip-width
apart, knees slightly bent. Face forward
with your arms hanging loosely by
your sides.

2. Rest your right hand on your left shoulder,
keeping your left arm soft and loose at
your side.

3. Engage your lower stomach muscles, then allow your left arm to
float up, feeling the movement through your fingers on your right hand.
When you feel your left shoulder lift under your hand, allow your arm
to lower to the starting position. Repeat the exercise with the opposite arm.

Muscles

Lengthen

Teres minor

Subscapularis

Infraspinatus

Strengthen

Lower trapezius

Serratus anterior

Deltoid

GOOD FOR:

Neck strain

Rotator cuff pain

Swimmer's
shoulder

Biceps tendonitis

Acromioclavicular
joint sprain

Common mistakes to avoid

Don't use your neck muscles to pull up the arm.

Don't allow your ribs to move during the arm raise. Keep your
core stable.

Don't allow your entire body to move with the movement
of your arm.

Four point challenge

SPORTS: ALL

Focus

To release and localize movement at the base of the spine

Breathe OUT as you curl your spine under. Breathe IN as you uncurl your spine.

Method

1. Kneel on all fours, with your hands placed directly beneath your shoulders. Your knees should be in line with your hips and the lower part of your legs straight. Keep your head parallel to the floor. Maintain the neutral curve in your spine while drawing your shoulder blades down your back. Keep your elbows soft and your weight equally balanced between your hands and knees.

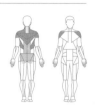

Muscles
Lengthen
Lumbar erector spinae
Gluteals

Strengthen
Lower abdominals
Scapular stabilizers
Latissimus dorsi

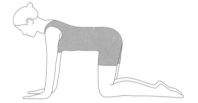 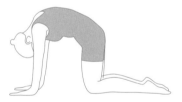

2. Move your focus to the base of your spine. Curl your tail bone under, slowly moving your focus up your spine, rounding the spine as you go.

3. When your focus reaches the top of your head, your back should be rounded, with your chin on your chest and your neck long. Breathe in and uncurl your spine.

Common mistakes to avoid

Don't shift your weight between your hands. Keep your weight evenly balanced.

Don't drop your head down or poke your chin out. Keep your neck stretched long and strong.

GOOD FOR:
Low-back pain
Shoulder injuries
Neck strain

Hip opening

SPORTS: BASEBALL, CYCLING, FOOTBALL, HOCKEY, RUNNING, SAILING, SKIING, SOCCER, SWIMMING, TENNIS

Focus

To improve activation of hip lateral rotation muscles
To move the hip joint without moving the pelvis

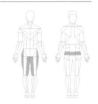

Breathe OUT as the top knee lifts. Breathe IN as the leg lowers.

Method

1. Lie on your side, knees bent and toes in line with your knees. Stretch your lower arm out above your head, so that it is in line with your body.

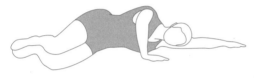

Muscles
Lengthen
Hip abductors
Tensor fasciae latae
Iliotibial band
Hip adductors

Strengthen
Gluteus medius
Transversus abdominis

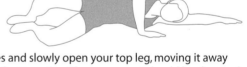

2. Engage your lower stomach muscles and slowly open your top leg, moving it away from the bottom one, keeping your feet together. The movement should be slow and controlled. Do not allow the lower back to move. Hold and lower, then repeat on the other side.

GOOD FOR:
Hip pain
Hamstring strain
Patellofemoral pain
Stress fracture
Achilles tendonitis
Ankle inversion injury
Plantar fasciitis

Common mistakes to avoid

Don't allow the waist to sink into the floor.

Keep your pelvis in the neutral position throughout the entire exercise.

Don't let your upper body roll forward.

Variations

This exercise can be made harder by extending your feet further from your body. This increases the lever length in the hip area (gluteus medius).

Pelvic stability

SPORTS: HOCKEY, RUNNING, SAILING, TENNIS

Focus

To keep the pelvis in a stable, neutral position while moving limbs

Method

1. Lie on your back with your feet hip-width apart, arms at your sides, shoulder blades drawn down the back. Check that your pelvis is in a neutral position, tailbone down and lengthening away. Place your hands on your pelvic bones to check for unwanted movement and to check that the lower abdominals stay scooped.

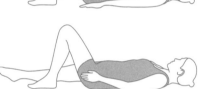

2. Test your pelvic stability by sliding one leg away along the floor. Keep the lower abdominals engaged and the pelvis still. Breathe into your lower rib-cage while you return the leg to the bent position, keeping the stomach hollow.

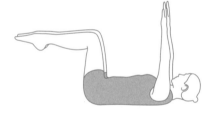

Muscles

Lengthen

Gluteals

Hamstrings

Erector spine

Strengthen

Tensor fasciae latae

Lower abdominals

Obliques

Abductors/adductors

GOOD FOR:

Low-back pain

Tronchanteric hip pain

Patellofemoral pain

Stress fracture

Achilles problems

Ankle inversion injury

Plantar fasciitis

Variation

Breathe in wide and full to prepare. Breathe out, zip up, and hollow and fold the right knee up. Think of the thigh bone dropped down into the hip and anchoring there. Do not lose your neutral pelvis, the tailbone stays down. Breathe in and hold. Breathe out, as you return the foot slowly to the floor.

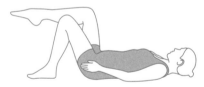

Imprinting

SPORTS: ALL

Focus

Become aware of the movement of the individual vertebrae in relation to one another

To produce very small movement of the vertebrae along the length of the spine

To release tension in and around the vertebrae

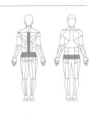

Muscles
Strengthen

Transversus abdominis

Multifidis.

**Breathe OUT as you imprint the spine.
Breathe IN as you release the imprint.**

Method.

1. Lie on your back in the neutral position (see opposite).

2. Slowly imprint each vertebra one by one into the floor, working from the bottom to the top and back again. Do not force the movement. If you're a beginner, concentrate on moving sections of the spine. As you become more advanced, these sections should become smaller.

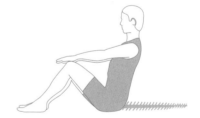

GOOD FOR:
Low-back pain

Common mistakes to avoid

Don't force or exaggerate the movement.

Make sure that you maintain your spine in a neutral position throughout.

Neutral spine

SPORTS: ALL

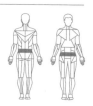

Focus
To correct alignment of the pelvis

Muscles
Strengthen
Transversus abdominis

Method

1. Lie on the floor, with your knees bent, feet hip-width apart. Your chest and ribs should be wide open and your shoulder blades slightly lengthened down your back. Your forehead should be parallel to the ceiling and your jaw relaxed.

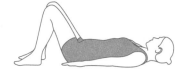

2. Gently and without discomfort, tilt your pelvis forward and backward. The middle area of this movement is the neutral position for your pelvis. Take care not to force the movement, as it takes time to adapt to this position.

GOOD FOR:
Low back pain
Patellofemoral pain
Hamstring strain

Common mistakes to avoid
Don't lock your lower back onto the floor and hold it while doing any exercises.

Don't give up if you can't get the position straight away. You may need to practice for some time to find your neutral position.

Static standing balance

SPORTS: ALL

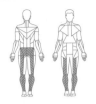

Focus

To maintain good alignment of the trunk while standing

To improve muscles, coordination in the lower limbs

Breathe normally throughout the exercise.

Muscles
Strengthen

Tibialis anterior

Tibialis posterior

Peroneus longus/brevis

Calf muscle

Quadriceps

Hamstrings

Gluteals

Core stability

Hip stabilizers

Method

1. Stand with your feet hip-width apart, hands hanging loosely by your sides. Your weight should be balanced evenly on your feet between your big toe, little toe, and heel.

2. Lift one leg off the floor, maintaining a level position with your pelvis. Don't allow the hip to drop to one side. Use your lower abdominals to control your balance. Test your balance by leaning forward, back and to either side.

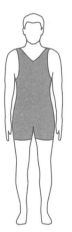
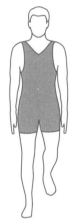

GOOD FOR:

All lower limb injuries

Common mistakes to avoid

Don't lose your balance.

Don't lose the neutral position of the pelvis.

Arm circles

SPORTS: BASEBALL, CYCLING, GOLF, SAILING, SKIING, SWIMMING, TENNIS

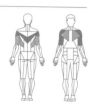

Focus

To enhance the muscles in the shoulders (scapular stabilizers)

To encourage ease of movement in the shoulder girdle

Breathe OUT as your raise your arms. Breathe IN as your arms return to your sides.

Muscles

Lengthen

Pectorals

Latissimus dorsi

Shoulder rotators
(internal/external)

Triceps

Method

1. Stand against a wall or about a foot away from it. Your feet should be hip-width apart. Lean against the wall with your knees bent. Imagine that you're sitting on a bar stool. Keep your pelvis in neutral and lengthen your body through the spine.

2. Engage your lower stomach muscles and reach your arms out in front of you, palms down. Raise your arms above your head, feeling your shoulder blades lengthen down your back as your arms float up.

3. Move your arms out to the sides and down in a continual arc (until they hang by your side).

Strengthen

Deltoid

Supraspinatus

Lower trapezius

Biceps

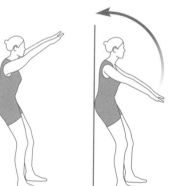

Common mistakes to avoid

Don't lose your neutral pelvis position during the movement.

Don't allow the ribs to lift when your raise your arms.

Don't restrict the movement with your shoulder blades as your raise your arms. Allow them to glide down your back.

Keep your neck long throughout the exercise.

Your elbows should be straight but not locked in at the elbow joint.

Only circle in a controlled range of movement, don't force it.

GOOD FOR:

Neck strain

Rotator cuff
pain

Biceps
tendonitis

179

Arm opening

SPORTS: BASEBALL, GOLF, HORSE RIDING, SAILING, SKIING, SOCCER, SWIMMING, TENNIS, WINDSURFING

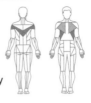

Focus
To open the front of the chest

To gently rotate through the upper thoracic spine for improved mobility

Breathe OUT as your arm opens the chest area.
Breathe IN as you return your arm to the starting position.

Muscles
Lengthen

Pectoralis minor

Method

1. Lie on your side with your head on a supporting pillow or towel. Bend your knees to a right angle to your body. Maintain a straight back with your pelvis in neutral. Extend your arms out in front of you, and draw your shoulder blades down your back.

Strengthen
Posterior deltoid
Rhomboids
Serratus anterior

2. Maintaining the length of your spine, extend and lift the top arm away from the bottom arm. Follow the movement of your hand with your head, keeping your chest open and your shoulder blades drawn down your back. Do not extend your upper arm further than the plane of your chest. This helps to avoid any strain on the anterior aspect of the shoulder joint.

GOOD FOR:

Rotator cuff pain

Acromioclavicular joint sprain

Shoulder dislocation

Muscle imbalance

3. Return your arm to the starting position.

Common mistakes to avoid
Don't push your arm beyond the line of your chest.

Don't lose the space between your shoulder and neck: keep the side of your neck open.

Big squeeze

SPORTS: BASEBALL, CYCLING, FOOTBALL, HORSE RIDING, RUNNING
SAILING, SWIMMING, TENNIS, WINDSURFING

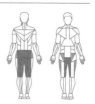

Focus

To engage the hamstrings

To enhance contraction of the gluteals

To stabilize the lumbar area

Breathe IN to prepare for the movement.
Breathe OUT as you squeeze the cushion.

Method

1. Lie on your front, with a narrow cushion between your thighs and
groin. Your feet should be turned out. Place your hands palms
down under your forehead, keeping your elbows wide and relaxed.

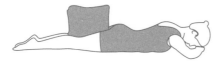

2. Engage your stomach muscle and gently squeeze the cushion
between your thighs. Hold this position.

Variation

From step 2, extend both feet off the floor about an inch and continue
to squeeze the cushion. Hold, maintaining the turned out feet position.
Don't lift your hips off the floor.

Muscles

Lengthen

Psoas

Tensor fasciae lata

Rectus abdominis

Abductors

Strengthen

Hamstrings

Gluteals

Adductors

GOOD FOR:

Patellofemoral knee
pain

Chondromalacia pain

Low-back pain

Common mistakes to avoid

Don't lose your core strength. Keep your back strong
and steady when you squeeze the cushion.

Don't allow your feet to turn in, keep them
turned outward.

Breathing patterns

SPORTS: ALL

Focus

To encourage the release of tension in the body

To allow your mind to focus on the movement

Method

1. Sitting or standing tall, wrap a band around your ribs, crossing it over at the front. Hold the ends of the band in your hands. Keep your shoulders relaxed, elbows open. Gently pull the band tight. Breathe in wide and allow your ribs to expand the material.

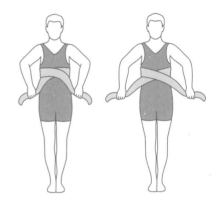

2. As you breathe out allow the breastbone to soften. Allow the ribs to slide down through the waist. If you need it, gently relax your grip on the material to allow your rib-cage to relax. Continue to breathe in and out in this way: practice this movement at least 10 times.

GOOD FOR:

All injuries

Common mistakes to avoid

Don't tense your shoulders.

Don't allow your breastbone to lift.

Don't breathe too quickly. Take natural breaths and stop if you become dizzy.

Dart

SPORTS: BASEBALL, CYCLING, GOLF, HORSE RIDING,
SAILING, SKIING, SOCCER, SWIMMING, TENNIS

Focus

To create awareness of the shoulder blades

To enhance the strength of the shoulder-blade muscles

To work the neck flexors

To strengthen the back extensor muscles

Breathe OUT at starting position and to engage the abdominal muscles. Breathe IN when raising your upper body.

Method

1. Lie on your front, with a flat pillow under your forehead to keep your neck open. Place your arms close to your sides, palms facing inward. Keep your legs together, with your toes parallel to the floor. Breathe in to prepare your body.

2. Breathe out, then engage the lower stomach muscles. Pull your shoulder blades down your back and lift your upper body off the floor, lengthening your fingers toward your feet. Keep your eyes focused downward and your head parallel to the floor.

3. Breathe in then lower your upper body slowly to the floor.

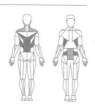

Muscles

Lengthen

Upper trapezius

Rectus abdominis

Pectoralis major and minor

Strengthen

Lower trapezius

Serratus anterior

Latissimus dorsi

Erector spinae

Lower abdominals

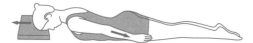

GOOD FOR:
Neck strain
Rotator cuff pain
Biceps tendonitis
Hamstring strain
Shoulder pain

Common mistakes to avoid

Don't allow your stomach muscle to slacken. Keep the lower stomach engaged during the exercise.

Don't tip your head back as you raise your head. This places a strain on your neck.

Don't allow your feet to raise off the ground.

Don't strain your lower back if you have forgotten to maintain the contraction in your lower stomach or risen too high for your level of control at this stage.

Hamstring lengthening

SPORTS: ALL

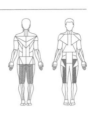

Focus

To achieve length in the hamstrings while maintaining a stable trunk.

Breathe OUT as you lengthen the leg away from you.
Breathe IN when returning the leg to starting position.

Muscles
Lengthen
Hamstrings
Adductors

Strengthen
Quadriceps
Hip flexors

Method

1. Lie on your back, feet hip-width apart and pelvis in neutral position. Bend your knees, resting your foot in a resistance band.

2. Push your foot away from your body, lengthening the leg as much as possible. Raise your leg up until you feel a pulling in the back of the leg. Be careful not to stretch the leg further than is comfortable. Hold this position for a couple of seconds, then lower the leg slowly. Repeat 10 times then change legs.

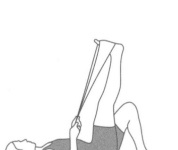

GOOD FOR:
Patellofemoral pain
Ankle inversion injury
Hamstring strain
Patellar tendonitis
Medial collateral ligament injury
Anterior cruciate ligament injury
Shin splints
Hip pain

Common mistakes to avoid

Don't overstretch the leg.

Be aware of the neutral position of your pelvis during the stretch.

Don't use your chest or spine to push the stretch.

Keep your legs parallel throughout the movement.

Long sitting stretch

SPORTS: BASEBALL, CYCLING, FOOTBALL, HOCKEY, HORSE RIDING, RUNNING, SAILING, SOCCER, SWIMMING, TENNIS

Focus

To stretch the lower and mid back

To stretch the adductors

Breathe OUT to lengthen away from the body. Breathe IN to return to the starting position.

Method

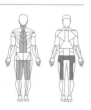

1. Sit evenly on the floor, sitting forward on your sitting bones. Rest one sole of your foot on the opposite calf, with the other leg straight out in front of you. Make sure you don't slump forward. Place a firm cushion under your bottom if necessary.

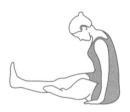

2. Curl your head down toward your chest bone. Imagine that there is a beach ball on your lap and you're bending your body over the ball. Use the arm on your bent leg side to support you, as you reach forward with the other arm. Alternate on both sides.

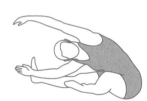

Variation

In the starting position, sit tall and raise your arms toward the ceiling, shoulder-width apart. Turn your body toward the bent knee, keeping the weight even on your sitting bones. Bend the arm on the bent-knee side, to try and lessen the area between the knee and armpit.

Common mistakes to avoid

Don't lose the even pressure on your sitting bones.

If you feel pain, stop pushing.

Don't allow the body to slump into the curl position.

Muscles

Lengthen

Hamstrings

Adductors

Lumbar spine

Erector spinae muscles

Strengthen

Lower abdominals

Soleus

Quadriceps

Rectus femoris

Deep neck flexors

GOOD FOR:

Hamstring strain
Patellofemoral pain
Ankle inversion
Achilles problems
Stress fracture
Low back strain

185

Mid-back stretch

SPORTS: BASEBALL, GOLF, FOOTBALL, HORSE RIDING,
SAILING, SKIING, SOCCER, SWIMMING, TENNIS

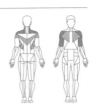

Focus
To lengthen the middle back muscles (mid trapezius and lower trapezius)

Breathe IN on the upward movement and OUT with the downward movement of the arms.

Muscles

Lengthen

Lower/mid trapezius

Posterior deltoid

Pectoralis major/minor

Latissimus dorsi

Subscapularis

Strengthen

Anterior deltoid

Biceps

Latissimus dorsi

Upper trapezius

Teres minor

Supraspinatus

Infraspinatus

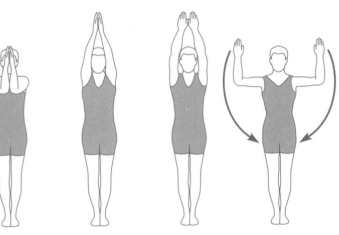

Method

1. Stand with your knees slightly bent, pelvis in neutral.

2. Place your elbows, forearms and palms together in front of your body. Keep the elbows tightly together as long as possible while raising the forearms over the face. Drop the forearms past the ears toward the floor, keeping the backs of the elbows open. Return your arms to your sides.

Common mistakes to avoid
Don't lose the stretch sensation by lowering your arms.

Don't lose the tightness throughout the motion.

> **GOOD FOR:**
>
> Rotator cuff pain
>
> Biceps tendonitis
>
> Acromioclavicular joint sprain

Neck rolls

SPORTS: BASEBALL, CYCLING, FOOTBALL, GOLF, SAILING,
SKIING, SOCCER, SWIMMING, TENNIS, WINDSURFING

Focus

To relax and release tension in the neck

To activate the deep neck flexors

Keep your normal breathing pattern.

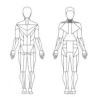

Muscles
Lengthen
Sternocleidomastoid

Strengthen
Deep neck flexors

Method

1. Lie on your back with your knees bent and your arms at your sides. Your neck should be long, resting on a small cushion. Keep your jaw relaxed and soft. To loosen the muscles turn your head slowly from side to side.

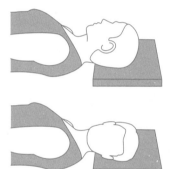

2. With the head in a central position, gently bow your head to bring the chin toward the chest, opening the back of the neck. Hold this position, making sure to keep your jawline soft. Allow the head to move back to the starting position.

GOOD FOR:

Neck strain
Shoulder pain

Common mistakes to avoid

Don't force the movement.

Don't rotate the head too far one way or another.

Don't lift your head from the cushion when tucking the chin in.

Roll downs

SPORTS: BASEBALL, CYCLING, FOOTBALL, GOLF, HOCKEY, RUNNING, SAILING, SKIING, SOCCER, SWIMMING, TENNIS, WINDSURFING

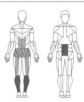

Focus

To engage the lower stomach muscles to control movement

To lengthen the hamstrings

Breathe IN to prepare. Breathe OUT to curl down and return to starting position.

Method

1. Stand tall, with your feet hip-width apart, knees slightly bent. Rest your arms at your side.

2. Engage your lower abdominals. Lower your chin to your chest and soften your chest bones as you curl forward. Allow your ribs to soften as you curl, but don't allow your posture to slump. Continue to engage your lower abdominals. When you have reached as far as you can, reverse the curl. Use your tailbone to pull downward in order to maintain the length of your spine and return you to the starting position.

Muscles

Lengthen

Hamstrings

Gluteals

Erector spinae

Hip rotators

Latissimus dorsi

Levator scapulae

Sternocleido mastoid

Neck extensors

Strengthen

Transversus abdominis

Soleus

Calf muscles

Gluteals

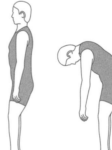
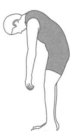
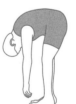

GOOD FOR:
Neck strain
Rotator cuff pain
Low-back strain
Ankle inversion injury
Hamstring strain
Tronchanteric hip pain

Common mistakes to avoid

Don't forget about your abdominals. Engage your lower abdominals throughout the entire movement.

Bend through your spine, not your hips.

Take care not to roll forward or to the side. Keep your weight evenly balanced on your feet.

Shoulder external rotation

SPORT: BASEBALL, CYCLING, FOOTBALL, GOLF, HOCKEY, SAILING, SKIING, SOCCER, SWIMMING, WINDSURFING

Focus

To control the shoulder blades as the upper arm moves

To strengthen the external rotation muscles

Breathe IN to prepare. Breathe OUT as your arm moves out to the side.

Method

1. Stand upright, with your shoulder blades drawn down your back, lower stomach muscles engaged and arms loosely at your sides.

2. Hold onto a resistance band that is not too tight to restrict the range of movement you can move through. Moving from the elbow, slowly pull your right hand out to the side, keeping your forearm parallel to the floor and your upper arm tight against your trunk. Hold this position, then slowly return to your arm to your side. Repeat on other arm.

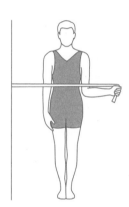

Muscles
Lengthen

Subscapularis

Strengthen

Infraspinatus

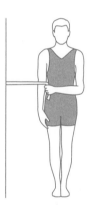

Common mistakes to avoid

Don't allow the trunk to move at the same time as the band is pulled out.

Don't move your elbow. Keep it tight against your body.

Don't rush it. The movement should be slow and controlled.

GOOD FOR:

Neck strain

Rotator cuff problems

Biceps tendonitis

Acromioclavicular joint sprain

Shoulder internal rotation

SPORTS: BASEBALL, CYCLING, FOOTBALL, GOLF, HOCKEY, SAILING, SKIING, SOCCER, SWIMMING, WINDSURFING

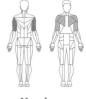

Focus

To control the stability of the shoulder blades as the upper arm moves

Breathe IN to prepare as the arm moves out.
Breathe OUT as the arm moves in.

Method

Muscles
Lengthen
Infraspinatus

Strengthen
Subscapularis

1. Attach a resistance band to a doorknob (door closed). Stand sideways to the door, shoulder blades drawn down your back. Your lower stomach muscles should be engaged.

2. Keeping your elbow tucked in to your side, slowly pull your hand toward your side. Your forearm should be parallel to the floor. Return to starting position.

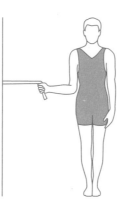
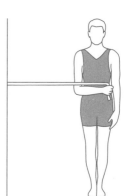

Common mistakes to avoid

Don't allow the trunk to move at the same time as the band is pulled out.

Don't move your arm. Keep your elbows tucked in at your side.

Don't jerk the band—make sure the movement is smooth.

GOOD FOR:

Neck strain
Rotator cuff pain
Biceps tendonitis
Acromioclavicular joint sprain

Shoulder push away

SPORTS: BASEBALL, CYCLING, FOOTBALL, GOLF, HOCKEY, SAILING, SKIING,
SOCCER, SWIMMING, WINDSURFING

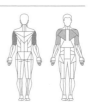

Focus

To control the movement of the anterior aspect of the shoulder

Breathe IN to prepare as the arm moves out.
Breathe OUT as the arm moves in.

Method

1. Stand or sit with your back to the door with a band fixed
at elbow height to a secure point such as a door handle. Your
elbow should be bent at 90 degrees parallel to the floor.

Muscles
Lengthen
Posterior aspect of the
deltoid

Teres minor

Triceps

Strengthen
Anterior deltoid

Pectoralis major/minor

Lower trapezius

Serratus anterior

Deep neck flexors

Biceps

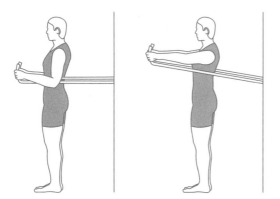

2. Push your hands forward, keeping the forearms
parallel to the floor as you push out. Return to the
starting position.

GOOD FOR:

Neck strain

Rotator cuff pain

Biceps tendonitis

Acromioclavicular
joint sprain

Common mistakes to avoid

Don't move your trunk. Keep your trunk and shoulders
stable as you push forward.

Shoulder rotation contro

SPORTS: BASEBALL, FOOTBALL, GOLF, HORSE RIDING, SAILING, SKIING,
SOCCER, SWIMMING, WINDSURFING

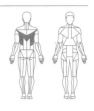

Focus

To enhance the full range of motion in the shoulder

To prevent compensating movements when rotating the shoulder

To prevent misuse of the scapular when rotating the shoulder

To improve flexibility in the shoulder rotator muscles

Muscles
Lengthen
Shoulder rotators

Strengthen
Shoulder rotators
Scapular stabilizers
Latissimus dorsi

Method

1. Lie on your back, with your knees bent and pelvis in neutral position. Bend your arms up to shoulder level, hands pointing to the ceiling.

2. Place your right hand on to your left shoulder. Move your left hand toward your head, feeling the push onto your resting hand. Continue until you feel a pulling sensation in your shoulder joint. Return to the starting position. Move the same hand toward your hip, again until you feel a pulling sensation in your shoulder joint. Return to the starting position and repeat on the other side.

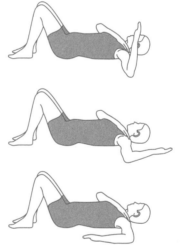

Common mistakes to avoid

Don't allow the shoulder to lift during the movement.

Don't allow the shoulder to drop or move toward the trunk

Don't lose your neutral position of the pelvis.

Don't stretch or strain your neck. Keep your neck soft and open during the exercise.

GOOD FOR:

Shoulder dislocation
Muscle imbalance
Biceps tendonitis
Rotator cuff pain
Acromioclavicular
joint sprain

Shoulder rowing

SPORTS: BASEBALL, FOOTBALL, GOLF, HORSE RIDING, SAILING, SOCCER, SWIMMING, TENNIS, WINDSURFING

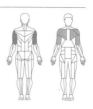

Focus

To control the movement of the posterior aspect of the shoulder

Method

1. Stand or sit facing a closed door, onto which a band is fixed at elbow height. Bend your elbow 90 degrees parallel to the floor.

2. Pull the left hand toward you. Keep the forearm parallel to the floor as you pull. Hold, then return to the starting position. Repeat with the other side.

Muscles

Lengthen

Anterior deltoid

Pectoralis minor

Biceps

Strengthen

Posterior deltoid

Infraspinatus

Triceps

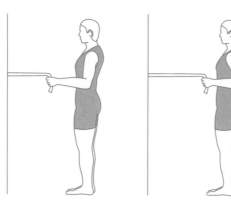

GOOD FOR:

Rotator cuff pain

Neck strain

Acromioclavicular joint sprain

Swimmer's shoulder

Common mistakes to avoid

Don't move your body or shoulder as you push forward. Keep your shoulder still throughout the exercise.

Side reach

SPORTS: BASEBALL, CYCLING, FOOTBALL, RUNNING, SAILING, SWIMMING, TENNIS

Focus
To lengthen through the whole side

Breathe IN to prepare. Breathe OUT to raise your arm and IN when returning to the starting position.

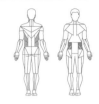

Muscles
Lengthen
Latissimus dorsi
Obliques
Side flexors in the neck

Method

1. Stand with your feet hip-width apart, with your hands loosely at your sides.

2. Slowly raise you arm above your head, while allowing the opposite arm to slide down your leg. Keep your raised arm in line with your body and avoid twisting your trunk. Stretch your arm as far as you can to open your side.

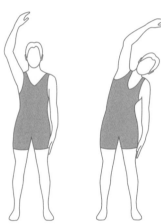

Strengthen
Obliques
Quadratus lumborum

GOOD FOR:

Low-back strain
Rotator cuff pain
Biceps tendonitis
Patellofemoral pain
Hamstring strain

Common mistakes to avoid
Don't twist your body when reaching.
Make sure that your arm is over your head not across the front of your body.

Single knee kicks

SPORTS: BASEBALL, CYCLING, FOOTBALL, GOLF, HORSE RIDING,
RUNNING, SAILING, SOCCER, SWIMMING

Focus

To lengthen through the front of the leg

To improve the action of the hamstrings

To improve control of the lumbar extensor and lumbar stabilizer muscles

To prevent an excessive collapse of the lumbar spine during movement

Breathe OUT as you bend the knee. Breathe IN as you straighten your knee.

Muscles

Lengthen

Quadriceps

Psoas

Tensor fasciae latae

Strengthen

Hamstrings

Hip extensors

Lower abdominals

Method

1. Lie face down with your legs slightly apart and rest your head in your hands. Engage your shoulder blades, gently pulling the blades down your spine. Keep your forehead parallel to the floor.

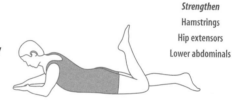

2. Bend your knee, so that your left foot touches your buttock. Point your foot slightly. Return to starting position. Repeat the movement with your foot flexed. Return to start position and repeat, alternating between pointing and flexing your foot. Swap sides and repeat.

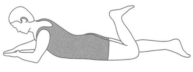

GOOD FOR:
Low back pain
Hip pain
Patellofemoral pain
Ankle inversion injury
Hamstring strain

Variation

Repeat the movement with your thigh slightly off the floor.

Common mistakes to avoid

Don't move your back during the exercise.

Don't poke your chin out.

Don't slump forward. Remain strong through the chest.

Be careful not to arch your back.

Spinal curls

SPORTS: BASEBALL, CYCLING, FOOTBALL, GOLF, HOCKEY, HORSE RIDING,
RUNNING, SAILING, SOCCER, SWIMMING, TENNIS

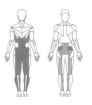

Focus

To enhance the segmental control in the lumbar spine

To lengthen the latissimus dorsi muscle

Breathe IN to prepare. Breathe OUT as you curl your spine up and float your arms up. Breathe IN at the hold point, then OUT as you return to neutral.

Muscles
Lengthen

Latissimus dorsi

Tibialis anterior

Rectus abdominis

Quadriceps

Psoas

Erector spinae

Method

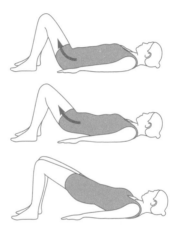

1. Lie on your back with your knees bent and feet flat on the floor, hip-width apart. Your arms should be loosely at your sides, shoulders wide and shoulder blades elongated down your spine.

2. Engage your lower abdominal muscles and slowly curl from the base of your spine. Allow each segment to curl, bit by bit, under and away from you. Hold the end position, then reverse the movement to return to the starting position. Repeat, aiming higher through the lumber spine. When you have reached your optimum movement, hold, and allow your shoulder blades to drift down your back. Raise your arms up, close to the sides of your head. Stop when your chest and ribs start to rise. Return your spine to neutral position by rolling your spine down. Allow your arms to float back to your sides.

Strengthen

Gluteus

Deep lumbar muscles

Erector spinae

Deep abdominals

Hamstrings

Adductors

Quadratus lumborum

Latissimus dorsi

Soleus

Common mistakes to avoid

Don't curl too high: keep your tailbone curled under.

Don't rest your weight on your shoulders.

Don't raise your arms too high. Your chest and ribs should stay on the floor.

GOOD FOR:

Low-back pain

Ankle inversion injury

Stress fracture

Hamstring strain

Tronchanteric hip pain

Shin splints

Standing Squat

SPORTS: BASEBALL, CYCLING, FOOTBALL, HOCKEY, RUNNING, SAILING,
SKIING, SOCCER, SWIMMING, TENNIS, WINDSURFING

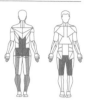

Focus

To keep the alignment of your lumbar spine throughout the movement

Breathe IN to prepare. Breathe OUT as you perform the movement.

Method

1. Using a resistance band suitable for your level, stand in a neutral position with your feet hip-width apart on the band. Wrap the ends of the band around your hands. Stretch the band until it's taut.

Muscles

Lengthen

Calf muscles

Hamstrings

Strengthen

Gluteus

Quadriceps

Adductors

Erector spinae

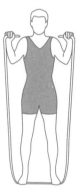

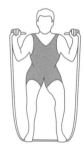

GOOD FOR:

Hip pain

Patellofemoral pain

Plantar fasciitis

Ankle inversion injury

Achilles tendonitis

Stress fracture

Hamstring strain

2. Engage your lower abdominals and slowly bend your knees, curling your pelvis under as you perform the squat. When your thighs are parallel to the floor, return to the starting position.

Common mistakes to avoid

Don't bend forward. Keep your spine aligned when squatting.

Star

SPORTS: BASEBALL, CYCLING, GOLF, HORSE RIDING, RUNNING, SAILING, SWIMMING, TENNIS, WINDSURFING

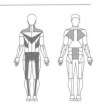

Focus

To stabilize the trunk using the extensor muscles of the back

To strengthen the gluteal muscles

To establish control of the center and core of the body

Breathe IN to prepare and OUT as your lift your arm and leg.

Method

1. Lie on your front with your feet hip-width apart, legs turned out from the hips. Place your arms above your head, wider than your shoulders. Place a pillow under your head for support.

2. Breathe out and engage the lower abdominal muscles. Raise your left arm an inch or so above the floor and hold. Then raise the opposite leg, lengthening away from your center. Make sure to keep your hips on the floor. Repeat on the opposite side.

Muscles
Lengthen

Upper trapezius

Rectus abdominis

Pectoralis major/minor

Strengthen

Lower abdominal muscles

Erector spinae

GOOD FOR:

Rotator cuff pain

Biceps tendonitis

Hamstring strain

Common mistakes to avoid

Don't twist your pelvis or trunk as your raise your leg.

Don't over-reach through the arms.

Don't lift your hips off the floor.

Keep your head down. Lifting it may cause damage in your neck.

T-band balance

SPORTS: ALL

Focus
To maintain good alignment of the trunk
To improve muscle coordination in the lower limbs

Before you start
Make sure that you're pain free when standing in neutral.
Do the hip opening exercise on page 174.

Breathe IN to prepare. Breathe OUT to stretch the band.

Method

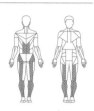

Muscle
Strengthen
Tibialis anterior/posterior
Peroneus longus/brevis
Calf muscles
Quadriceps
Hamstrings
Hip stabilizers

1. Stand upright, feet hip-width apart. Ground one foot firmly, with your weight balanced evenly between the toes and heel. Under the other foot, place a resistance band around your ankle and pick up any slack.

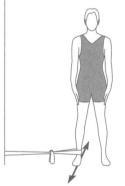
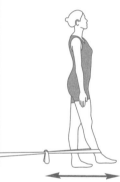

2. Pull the band either behind the leg or swap sides. Continue until the leg feels tired.

GOOD FOR:	
Ankle inversion injury	Shin splints
Patellofemoral pain	Calf strain
Patellar tendonitis	Meniscus tear
Achilles tendonitis	Stress fracture
Soccer ankle	Plantar fasciitis

Common mistakes to avoid
Don't lose your balance.

Don't lose your alignment.

Don't let band fall from your foot. Make sure that the band is secured properly.

Threading the needle

SPORTS: BASEBALL, CYCLING, GOLF, HORSE RIDING, SAILING, SKIING, SOCCER, SWIMMING, TENNIS

FOCUS
To achieve rotation in the thoracic spine

Breathe IN to prepare yourself. Breathe OUT as you reach through.

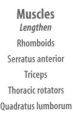

Method

1. Kneel on all fours, with your hands under your shoulders, knees level with your hips. Your spine should be in a neutral position.

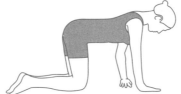

2. Engage the lower abdominals. Stretch your right arm through, under your trunk, to the opposite side until it is level with your shoulder. Drop your supporting elbow to the floor as you reach. Bring your ear to the floor and push your arm through until you feel the stretch in your thoracic spine. Return to the starting position and repeat on the opposite side.

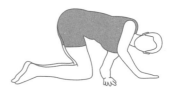

Muscles

Lengthen
Rhomboids
Serratus anterior
Triceps
Thoracic rotators
Quadratus lumborum

Strengthen
Latissimus dorsi
Biceps
Deltoid
Thoracic rotators

GOOD FOR:

Neck strain
Low-back pain
Rotator cuff pain
Biceps tendonitis
Acromioclavicular joint sprain

Common mistakes to avoid

Don't forget to bend the elbow on the weight-bearing arm as you reach through.

Don't release the movement too early. Keep stretching until you feel the reach in your spine.

Don't strain your neck. Lower your head to the floor as far as you can.

Wall slides

SPORTS: BASEBALL, CYCLING, FOOTBALL, GOLF, HOCKEY, RUNNING, SAILING, SKIING, SOCCER, TENNIS, WINDSURFING

Focus

To maintain alignment in the lower limbs during the exercise

To enhance the contraction of the knee stabilizer muscles

To maintain a neutral pelvis during the exercise

Breathe IN to prepare. Breathe OUT as you slide down the wall. Breathe IN as you hold, then OUT as you slide up.

Muscles

Lengthen

Calf muscles

Hamstrings

Gluteals

Strengthen

Quadriceps

Hip flexors

Calf muscles

Method

1. Stand against the wall, with your feet a foot-length from the wall, knees hip-width apart. Keep your feet evenly balanced on the floor.

2. Slide your back down the wall, keeping your knees parallel. Your kneecap should be over the second toe. Be careful not to let the foot roll out or to drop your knees. Hold this position and push through your knees to return to starting position.

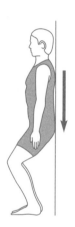

Common mistakes to avoid

Don't lose the neutral pelvis. Continue to keep your trunk engaged and connected to your body.

Don't allow your knees to drop to one side.

Make sure your feet remain in a balanced position.

GOOD FOR:		
Patellofemoral pain	Anterior cruciate ligament injury	Stress fracture
Patellar tendonitis	Shin splints	Achilles tendonitis
Hamstring strain	Ankle inversion injury	Plantar fasciitis
Medial collateral ligament damage	Soccer ankle	Low-back strain
	Calf strain	Swimmer's knee
		Swimmer's ankle

Windows

SPORTS: BASEBALL, CYCLING, FOOTBALL, GOLF, HORSE RIDING,
SAILING, SKIING, SOCCER, SWIMMING, TENNIS

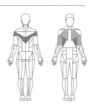

Focus
To open up the anterior chest muscles

**Breathe IN to prepare. Breathe OUT as the arms open.
Breathe IN as the arms return to the starting position.**

Muscles
Lengthen

Pectoralis major

Biceps

Subscapularis

Strengthen

Posterior deltoid

Infraspinatus

Scapular stabilizing
muscles

Method

1. Stand in neutral
position, feet
hip-width apart,
your elbows raised
in front of your body
and your upper
arms parallel to the
floor. Pull your
shoulder blades
down your spine.

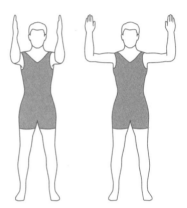

2. Engage your lower abdominals and pull your elbows
out so that your chest is wide. Keep your shoulders and
trunk stable: don't allow your back to arch or move.
Return your forearms to the starting position.

GOOD FOR:

Neck strain
Biceps tendonitis
Rotator cuff pain
Acromioclavicular
joint sprain

Common mistakes to avoid
Don't arch through your back.

Make sure that your forearms are parallel to your body and
your upper arms parallel to the floor.

Don't force the movement .

Wrist openings

SPORTS: CYCLING, FOOTBALL, GOLF, SAILING, SWIMMING, TENNIS, WINDSURFING

Focus
To localize movement in the forearms

Breathe IN to prepare. Breathe OUT when you open your hands.

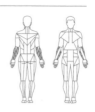

Muscles
Strengthen

Forearm flexors

Forearm extensors

Method

1. Sit with your elbows bent at 90 degrees. Keep your elbows tight at your sides. Make sure the backs of your hands and your forearms are in a straight line with the middle knuckle. The palms should be facing the body.

2. Slowly and in a controlled manner open and close your hands, without allowing it to lose its position.

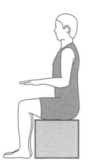

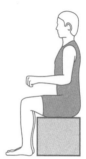

Variation
Increase the speed of movement.

GOOD FOR:
Shoulder pain
Tennis elbow
Biceps tendonitis
Golfer's elbow

Common mistakes to avoid
Don't allow your head to move. Keep it steady throughout the movement.

Don't rush. The movement should be slow and controlled.

Don't move your hand. Keep it level throughout the exercise.

Bridging

SPORTS: BASEBALL, CYCLING, FOOTBALL, GOLF, HOCKEY, HORSE RIDING, RUNNING, SKIING, SAILING, SOCCER, SWIMMING, TENNIS, WINDSURFING

Focus

To maintain trunk stability

To strengthen the gluteus and hamstrings

Breathe IN to prepare. Breathe OUT to raise your trunk, and IN as you lower.

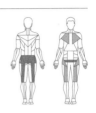

Muscles

Lengthen

Quadriceps

Hip flexors (psoas, tensor fasciae latae)

Pectoralis major/minor

Method

1. Lie on your back in the neutral position, arms at your sides, knees bent. Engage the lower abdominals, and push through your feet, engaging your gluteals as you do so.

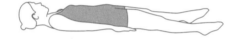

Strengthen

Gluteus

Hamstrings

Lower abdominals

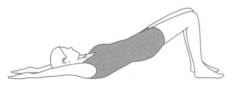

2. Engage your hips and lift your lower body, keeping your spine level. Lift your arms above your head, making sure to keep your ribs stable. Use your abdominals to bring your pelvis back to neutral. Return your arms to your sides.

Variation

Maintain the bridge and level pelvis position. Lift your right leg, raising your foot to the ceiling in a controlled way.

Common mistakes to avoid

Don't push too hard as this will create stress on your neck.

Make sure you use your gluteals to hold the raised position.

Maintain a neutral position as your raise your lower body.

GOOD FOR:	
Low-back pain	Anterior cruciate ligament problems
General knee pain	Plantar fasciitis
Ankle inversion injury	Patellofemoral pain
Meniscus tear	Spondylolisthesis
Hamstring strain	Piriformis pain
Achilles tendonitis	Gluteal hip pain
Medial collateral ligament pain	Adductor strain

Double leg stretch

SPORTS: BASEBALL, CYCLING, FOOTBALL, GOLF, HOCKEY, HORSE RIDING, RUNNING, SAILING, SKIING, SWIMMING, TENNIS, WINDSURFING

Focus

To strengthen the abdominals while moving the center of gravity

To strengthen the deep neck flexors

To coordinate your breathing throughout the sequence

Breathe IN to prepare. Breathe OUT as you stretch your arms and legs away from the starting position. Breathe IN as you return to the starting position.

Muscles
Lengthen

Latissimus dorsi

Pectoralis major/minor

Method

1. Lie on your back with your knees on your chest. Hold your knees with your hands, knees hip-width apart, big toes together.

Strengthen

Abdominals

Deep neck flexors

Adductors

Psoas

Latissimus dorsi

Lower trapezius

Gluteus medius

External hip rotators

2. Slowly curl your upper trunk to lengthen and lift the back of your neck. Straighten your legs, so that they are turned out from the hips, heels together. Flex your feet and feel your legs lengthen through the heels. Take your arms up into a wide sweep, until they are level with your ears. Circle your arms back around to your thighs. Lower your head to the starting position and bend your knees.

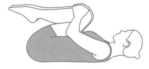

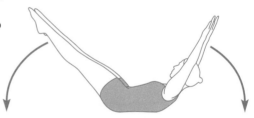

Common mistakes to avoid

Don't let your abdominals relax during the exercise.

Don't poke your neck out during the exercise.

Don't take your arms beyond your ears. This will cause your rib cage to rise and lose control over your trunk.

GOOD FOR:	
Shoulder dislocation	Golfer's elbow
Hamstring strain	Neck strain
Low-back pain	Acromioclavicular joint pain
Piriformis syndrome	Muscle imbalance
Gluteal hip pain	Patellofemoral pain
Achilles tendonitis	Patellar tendonitis
Anterior knee pain	Shoulder pain

Eccentric hamstrings

SPORTS: BASEBALL, FOOTBALL, RUNNING, SKIING, SOCCER, TENNIS

Focus

To strengthen your hamstrings

To enhance contraction of the hamstrings

To prevent injury to your hamstrings

Breathe OUT to extend your knee.
Breathe IN to bend your knee.

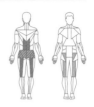

Method

1. Lie on your stomach on a bed, so that your head and shoulders are lower than your waist and hips. Your legs should have the ability to straighten without limitation.

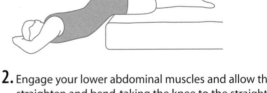

2. Engage your lower abdominal muscles and allow the knee to straighten and bend, taking the knee to the straightened position before repeating the bend. Continue bending and straightening your knee, increasing the speed as you go.

Common mistakes to avoid

Don't do too many reps as this can lead to muscle soreness.

Make sure you extend your leg out completely before bending it again.

Don't move your hips. Keep your hips neutral as the knee bends.

Don't let your hips raise as you bend your knees.

Muscles

Lengthen

Hip flexors

Psoas

Quadriceps

Gluteals

Strengthen

Hamstrings

GOOD FOR:

Hamstring strain

Medial collateral ligament injury

Anterior cruciate ligament injury

Patellofemoral pain

Hip pain

Gluteal hip pain

Heel drop

SPORTS: CYCLING, GOLF, RUNNING, SKIING, SOCCER, TENNIS

Focus

To allow the development of the eccentric muscle contraction of the Achilles complex (gastrocnemius/soleus)

Method

1. Stand in alignment, with both heels over the edge of a step or a raise.

Muscles
Strengthen and lengthen

Eccentric to
Gastrocnemius

Soleus

Tibialis anterior/posterior

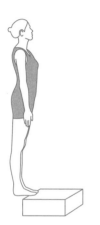
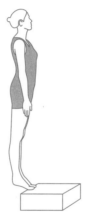
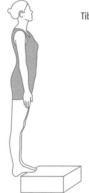

2. Raise up on your toes, then allow your heels to drop over the edge. The movement should be slow and controlled. Try this movement with your knees straight and your knees bent. Do a maximum three sets of 15 reps on alternate days. If you experience pain, don't progress to the next stage until you are pain-free. Apply local ice after each block of exercise.

Common mistakes to avoid

Don't progress too quickly. Take your time moving up to the next stage. Stop if you feel any pain.

Maintain your alignment throughout.

GOOD FOR:

Achilles tendonitis

Ankle inversion injury

Groin injury

Hundred

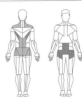

Focus

To strengthen the abdominal muscles

To coordinate your breathing

Breathe OUT using the abdominal muscles. Breathe IN wide and full through the ribs.

Method

1. Lie on your back with your knees bent at 90 degrees. Knees should be hip-width apart, toes pressed together. Reach your arms straight upward, palms facing forward.

2. Reach your arms down to the floor but don't rest your palms on the floor. Curl your head up and roll up through your abdominals so that your shoulders are just off the floor. Depending on your level, either keep your knees bent, or, if you're more practiced lengthen your feet away from you until they are straight. The whole leg should be turned out from your hips, with your heels touching. Tap the floor with your palms, exhaling to the count of five beats, inhaling to the count of five.

Common mistakes to avoid

Don't lose control of your lower abdominals. Lower back pain may be caused by weak abdominals.

Don't lose your neutral pelvis position.

Don't place any strain in your neck.

Don't move your trunk when you beat your arms.

Muscles

Lengthen

Erector spinae

Upper trapezius

Gluteals

Strengthen

Rectus abdominis

Obliques

Psoas

Lower trapezius

Deep neck flexors

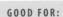

GOOD FOR:	
Rotator cuff pain	Hamstring strain
Golfer's elbow	Achilles tendonitis
Neck strain	Gluteal hip pain
Acromioclavicular joint pain	Piriformis pain
Shoulder dislocation	Calf muscle strain
Low-back pain	Groin injuries
Patellofemoral pain	Biceps tendonitis
Shoulder dislocation	Muscle imbalance

Knee/leg circles

SPORTS: FOOTBALL, GOLF, SOCCER

Focus

To move the leg independently of the hip joint

To challenge the stability of the lumbar spine

To maintain control of the neutral pelvis

Breathe OUT as you circle your leg outward.
Breathe IN as you circle the leg in.

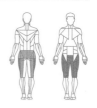

Muscles

Lengthen

Gluteals

Hip lateral rotators

Hamstrings

Strengthen

Psoas

Rectus femoris

Lower abdominals

Hip adductors/abductors

Method

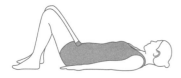

1. Lie with your knees bent, feet hip-width apart, shoulder blades drawn down your back, arms at your sides.

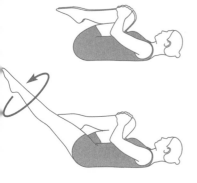

2. Engage your lower stomach muscles and fold both knees up to your chest. Keep one knee in this position and allow the other leg to rotate in the hip joint and open your knee out as far as you can. Close your knees together, then repeat the circle.

Variations

Straighten one leg and repeat the circular movement with that leg. The size of the circle depends upon the amount of pelvic control you have.

GOOD FOR:

Low back pain

Hamstring strain

Medial collateral ligament

Anterior cruciate ligament

Common mistakes to avoid

Don't lose your neutral pelvis position during the exercise.

Maintain a soft chest during the exercise and don't tighten the ribs as your leg is moving.

Don't relax your stomach muscles while your legs are away from the body. Keep them engaged.

Lean forward bending

SPORTS: BASEBALL, CYCLING, FOOTBALL, HOCKEY, HORSE RIDING,
RUNNING, SAILING, SOCCER, TENNIS, WINDSURFING

Focus

To control the flexibility of the lumbar spine in relation to the movement of the hips

To increase flexibility in the hips

To reduce back strain

To increase the contraction of the gluteal muscles

Breathe OUT as you bend. Breathe IN when you return to the standing position.

Muscle

Lengthen

Gluteals

Soleus

Gastrocnemius

Hamstrings

Strengthen

Lumbar extensors

Lower abdominals

Gluteals

Method

1. Stand tall with your feet hip-width apart, pelvis in neutral.

2. Bend from your hips, sticking your bottom out and maintaining a straight spine. To return to neutral, tighten your gluteals and move throughout your hips to return to the standing position.

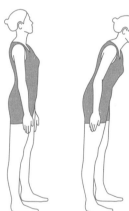
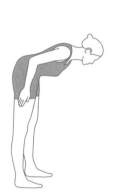

GOOD FOR:
Ankle inversion injury
Low-back pain
Patellofemoral pain
Hamstring strain
Groin injury

Common mistakes to avoid

Don't allow your back to bend.

Don't arch your back as you move forward.

Don't sway your back as you move through the range.

Leg pull back

SPORTS: BASEBALL, FOOTBALL, GOLF, HORSE RIDING,
SAILING, SKIING, SOCCER, WINDSURFING

Focus

To create stability in the shoulder girdle and upper arms

To stretch the hamstrings

To achieve mobility of the hips

Breathe OUT as you kick your legs out. Breathe IN as your leg lowers to the starting position.

Method

1. Sit on the floor with your legs extended in front of you and your hands pressed into the floor next to your buttocks. Contract your abdominals as you exhale and press into your palms, straightening your arms and body, lifting your hips and pointing your toes into the floor. Your forehead, shoulders, hips, and heels should form a straight line. Make sure your shoulder blades are pushed back and low down your back, so that your chest is open and your neck is long.

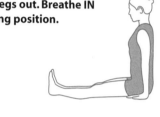

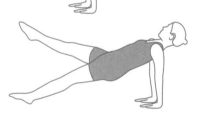

Muscles
Lengthen

Hamstrings

Psoas

Quadriceps

Strengthen

Shoulder muscles/scapular stabilizers

Foot muscles

Erector spinae

Latissimus dorsi

Anterior deltoid

2. Raise your right leg up, keeping your trunk and hips in neutral. Slowly lower your leg. Switch legs and repeat. When you've finished lower your body to the starting position.

Common mistakes to avoid

Don't relax your abdominals during the movement. Keep them contracted throughout.

Keep your legs as straight as possible.

Don't lose your neutral position during the exercise. Don't lock your elbows.

GOOD FOR:

Hamstring strain

Medial collateral ligament injury

Anterior cruciate ligament injury

Low back pain

Neck strain

Adductor strain

Spondylolisthesis

Leg pull prone

SPORT: BASEBALL, CYCLING, FOOTBALL, GOLF, RUNNING, SAILING,
    SKIING, SOCCER, SWIMMING, TENNIS, WINDSURFING

Focus

To control hip extension through the trunk

To create strength in the trunk and maintain upper-body control

To strengthen gluteus (buttock and thigh muscles)

Breathe OUT as your raise your leg. Breathe IN as the leg is lowered.

Method

1. Lie flat on your stomach with your legs hip width apart.
Your toes should be on the mat and palms directly under your shoulders.

2. Straighten your arms to raise your body into a push-up position. Hold your trunk and back in a straight line. Push through one foot while lifting the opposite leg. Alternate legs, keeping pressure through the heels.

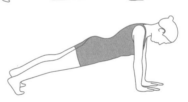

Variations

Repeat the push up, resting on your forearms instead of your hands.

Common mistakes to avoid

Don't lose your center or drop your hips.

Don't bend your elbows, keep them straight and strong.

Don't tense your shoulders.

Don't allow the raised leg to bend. Maintain a steady pressure in the heel.

Muscles

Lengthen

Quadriceps

Soleus

Rectus abdominis

Quadratus lumborum

Strengthen

Hip extensors

Hamstrings

Serratus anterior

Lower trapezius

Latissimus dorsi

Deep neck flexors

Pectoralis major/minor

Obliques

GOOD FOR:	
Meniscus tear	Medial collateral ligament injury
Low-back pain	Anterior cruciate ligament injury
Hamstring strain	
Swimmer's shoulder	Neck strain
Swimmer's elbow	Acromioclavicular joint sprain
Shoulder dislocation	
Spondylolisthesis	Shoulder pain
Biceps tendonitis	Sciatica

Lunge

SPORTS: BASEBALL, CYCLING, FOOTBALL, GOLF, HOCKEY, RUNNING, SAILING, SOCCER, SWIMMING, TENNIS, WINDSURFING

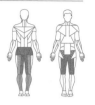

Focus

To strengthen the gluteals

To improve coordination of hip flexors in the lengthened position

Method

1. Stand in the neutral position, with your feet hip-width apart.

2. Take a comfortable step forward, keeping your trunk well aligned. Bend your front leg, so that the thigh is slightly below parallel. Return the legs to the starting position by pushing through the front foot.

Muscles

Lengthen

Hamstrings

Calf muscles

Hip flexors

Strengthen

Gluteals

Psoas

Quadriceps

Adductors

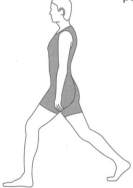

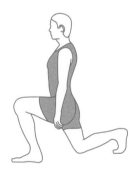

Variations

Increase the stride length.

Hold weights in your hands when you step forward.

Common mistakes to avoid

Don't allow your trunk to bend or slump forward.

Don't allow your trunk to twist as you step forward.

GOOD FOR:	
Ankle inversion injury	Patellofemoral pain
Low-back pain	Patellar tendonitis
Hamstring strain	Shin splints
Spondylolisthesis	Hip pain
Swimmer's knee	Gluteal hip pain

Mermaid

SPORTS: BASEBALL, FOOTBALL, GOLF, HOCKEY, HORSE RIDING, SAILING, SKIING, SOCCER, SWIMMING, TENNIS, WINDSURFING

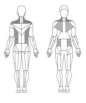

Focus

To stretch the side abdominals and the trunk muscles (quadratus lumborum)

To enhance the lengthening sensation in the lower back and chest

Breathe OUT as you engage your lower abdominal muscles and rotate. Breathe IN as you reach up.

Method

1. Sit on your hip, with your knee bent and your legs folded on top of each other and facing behind you.

2. Place your elbow on the mat beside you. At the same time, stretch the opposite arm overhead as far as you can reach.

3. Reverse the direction of the stretch and reach your arm to the opposite direction. Remember to keep your lower abdominals engaged. Repeat the movement on the opposite side.

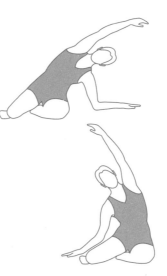

Muscles

Strengthen

Abdominals

Latissimus dorsi

Upper aspect of trapezius

Lengthen

Obliques

Quadratus lumborum

Latissimus dorsi

Serratus anterior

Pectoralis major/minor

GOOD FOR:

Shoulder impingement

Shoulder dislocation

Low-back pain

Shoulder pain

Acromioclavicular joint sprain

Rotator cuff pain

Muscle imbalance

Swimmer's shoulder

Spondylolisthesis

Variation

While reaching upward, arch your back and stretch your arm back as far as you can. Enhance this stretch by making a wide circle with your arm. Stretch your arm in front of you, so that your back is in a rounded position.

Common mistakes to avoid

Not reaching high enough to open the side of your chest.

If you experience any pain in your knees then sit on a pillow.

Oblique curl up

SPORTS: FOOTBALL, HOCKEY, HORSE RIDING, SOCCER, TENNIS, WINDSURFING

Focus

To strengthen the obliques

Breathe OUT to curl up. Breathe IN to curl down.

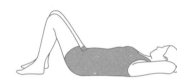

Method

1. Lie on the floor with your knees up, feet hip-width apart. Your hands should be behind your head, elbows open.

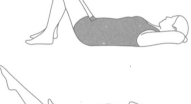

Muscles

Lengthen

Obliques

Quadratus lumborum

Strengthen

Obliques

Lower abdominals

2. Engage your lower stomach muscles and draw up your right shoulder towards your opposite knee. Your chest should be aimed toward your knee. Keep your elbow open and don't point it toward your knee. Continue the curl up until both your shoulder blades are off the floor. Hold this position, then lower your upper body slowly to the floor. Repeat on the other side.

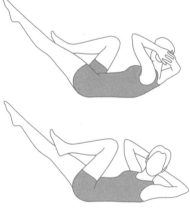

Variations

Repeat step one but pull your knees up to your chest. As you curl up towards the opposite knee, extend and straighten the other leg.

GOOD FOR:

Hamstring strain
Low-back pain
Groin injury
Adductor strain

Common mistakes to avoid

Don't lead the movement with your elbow.

Don't place any strain on your neck by pulling it forward.

Don't allow your trunk or pelvis to move toward your head as you curl up.

Open leg rocker

SPORTS: BASEBALL, CYCLING, FOOTBALL, HOCKEY, HORSE RIDING, RUNNING, SAILING, SKIING, SOCCER, SWIMMING

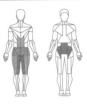

Focus

To enhance balance through the spine

To achieve maximum hamstring length

To achieve abdominal control

Breathe IN as you extend your legs. Breathe OUT as you roll back. Breathe IN as you roll upright.

Method

1. Sit with your knees bent, toes pointed and resting on the floor. Balance on your tailbone and straighten your legs into the air to form a V-shape.

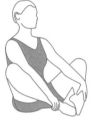

2. Slowly, with control, sink into your hips and curve your back into a C-shape, rolling along your spine until you reach your shoulders. Roll back to the upright position. Check to make sure your spine is aligned and your neck is long.

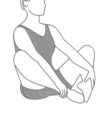

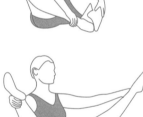

Muscles

Lengthen

Hamstrings

Gluteals

Strengthen

Gluteals

Hip abductors

Psoas

Rectus abdominis

Obliques

GOOD FOR:		
Patellofemoral pain	Ankle inversion injury	Stress fracture
Meniscus tear		Low-back pain
Hamstring strain	Medial collateral ligament injury	Patella tendonitis
Gluteal hip pain		Adductor strain
Calf muscle strain	Anterior cruciate ligament injury	
Swimmer's knee	Shin splints	

Common mistakes to avoid

Don't roll back farther than your shoulders to avoid neck strain.

If you feel unbalanced while rolling, bend your knees.

Don't slump your shoulders or abdominals.

Pilates Push–up

SPORTS: BASEBALL, CYCLING, FOOTBALL, GOLF, SAILING, SKIING, SWIMMING, TENNIS, WINDSURFING

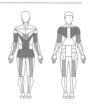

Focus

To strengthen the shoulder muscles

To achieve coordination of your shoulders and trunk

To activate the deep neck flexors

Breathe IN to prepare and as you walk your hands forward.
Breathe OUT as you roll down and bend your elbows.

Method

1. Stand with your shoulders relaxed, feet hip-width apart. Begin a roll down (see page 188) until your hands reach the floor. If you experience any tightness in your back, slightly bend your knees. When your hands reach the floor, walk your hands forward until they are aligned with your shoulders. Your body should be in a straight line, with your head down and shoulder blades drawn back.

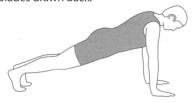

2. Bend your elbows and allow your body to move down to the floor, making sure to keep your trunk aligned. Hold this position and push your chest away from the floor. Reverse the movement and return to standing.

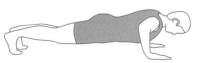

Muscles

Lengthen

Biceps

Rhomboids

Forearm extensors

Quadriceps

Hamstrings

Strengthen

Serratus anterior

Scapular stabilizers

Biceps

Pectoralis major

Anterior deltoid

Triceps

Lower abdominals

Gluteals

Back extensors

Common mistakes to avoid

Keep your body straight.

Don't arch your mid-back.

Don't move your hands forward. Keep them under your shoulders.

GOOD FOR:	
Shoulder dislocation	Biceps tendonitis
Neck strain	Muscle imbalance
Swimmer's elbow	Low-back pain
Swimmer's shoulder	Acromioclavicular joint sprain
Tennis elbow	Muscle imbalance

Praying mantis

SPORTS: BASEBALL, CYCLING, FOOTBALL, HOCKEY, HORSE RIDING, RUNNING, SAILING, SWIMMING, TENNIS, WINDSURFING

Focus

To establish coordination between the arms and a stable trunk

To improve the strength of the trunk muscles

To strengthen the scapular muscles

Breathe IN to prepare. Breathe OUT to engage abdominals and commence movement.

Muscles

Lengthen

Latissimus dorsi

Hip flexors

Biceps

Strengthen

Abdominals

Erector spinae

Gluteals

Scapular stabilizers

Triceps

Method

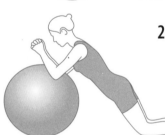

1. Kneel at the side of a fitness ball. Place your elbows on the ball with your hands clasped together. Engage your lower abdominal muscles and maintain a long spine.

2. Slowly, roll the ball forward with your elbows, taking care to keep your trunk controlled. Once you've pushed forward as far as you can, hold this position. Engage the lower abdominal muscles and return to the starting position. Repeat.

GOOD FOR:	
Low-back pain	Piriformis pain
Acromioclavicular joint pain	Gluteal hip pain
Spondylolisthesis	Hip pain
Shoulder pain	Hamstring strain
Shoulder dislocation	Neck strain

Common mistakes to avoid

Don't lose control of the ball. Work within comfortable boundaries.

Don't stick your gluteals out: maintain a neutral pelvis.

Don't allow your shoulders to lift up.

Roll up

Focus

To strengthen abdominals

To restore normal timing in lumbar flexion

To lengthen hamstrings

Breathe IN to prepare. Breathe OUT on the roll up. Breathe IN when you are in the stretched position. Breathe OUT when you return to the start position.

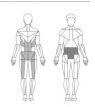

Muscles

Lengthen

Back extensors

Latissimus dorsi

Gluteals

Hamstrings

Method

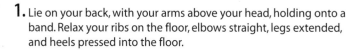

1. Lie on your back, with your arms above your head, holding onto a band. Relax your ribs on the floor, elbows straight, legs extended, and heels pressed into the floor.

2. Engage the lower stomach muscles to create a slight tension in your hip abductors. Stretch your arms out above your head and, imagining that someone is pulling on the band, begin to roll up. Continue to roll up, until your hands reach a point above your feet. Reverse the movement, keeping your stomach muscles engaged until your shoulder blades reach the floor and your arms return to the same point above your head. Lower your head to complete the movement.

Strengthen

Abdominals

Rectus abdominus

Obliques

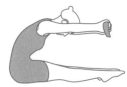

Common mistakes to avoid

Don't lose control of the lower abdominals.

Don't poke your chin upward. Imagine that there is a small orange under your chin that you don't want to lose.

Don't lift your legs off the floor.

Don't allow the band to drop. It has to act as a pulling mechanism throughout the movement.

Don't flop your body back onto the floor. The return movement should be slow and controlled.

GOOD FOR:	
Swimmer's knee	Shin splints
Patellofemoral pain	Stress fracture
Meniscus tear	Piriformis pain
Calf muscle strain	Gluteal hip pain

Rolling like a ball

SPORTS: CYCLING, FOOTBALL, GOLF, HOCKEY, HORSE RIDING, SWIMMING

Focus

To reduce tension in your spine

To gain and maintain control of balance point

To establish control of momentum of movement

Breathe IN to prepare. Breathe OUT as you begin the movement. Breathe IN as you return.

Method

1. Sit at the edge of your mat. Establish your balance point. Bend your knees until your feet touch your buttocks. Place your hands around the fronts of your knees.

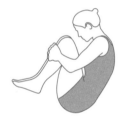 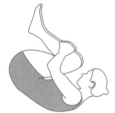 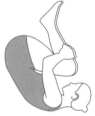

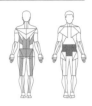

muscles
Lengthen
Erector spinae
Obliques
Hip abductors
Quadriceps
Quadratus lumborum
Latissimus dorsi

Strengthen
Lower abdominals
Rectus abdominis
Obliques
Quadratus lumborum
Hip adductors

2. Tuck your chin into your chest and contract your lower abdominal muscles. Allow your body to fall backward, bringing your legs with you. Keep your elbows wide. As you roll back maintain the distance between your chest and your thighs and keep your abdominals contracted. Make sure you keep your heels close to your buttocks. Allow your body to roll back to the starting position, using your glutes to help create momentum.

GOOD FOR:
Low-back pain
Hamstring strain
Spondylolisthesis
Ankle inversion injury
Knee injuries
Shoulder pain
Meniscus tear

Variation

Repeat the movement, but do so slowly, moving through each vertebra as you roll down and on your return. Don't jar your body.

Common mistakes to avoid

Don't relax your abdominals at any time during the movement. Keep them strong.

Don't roll back too far and place stress on your neck.

Scissors

SPORTS: BASEBALL, CYCLING, FOOTBALL, GOLF, HOCKEY, HORSE RIDING, RUNNING, SAILING, SKIING, SOCCER, TENNIS, WINDSURFING

Focus

To increase abdominal control

To stretch the upper back and neck

To mobilize the hips

To stretch the hip flexors

Breathe OUT as the legs open. Breathe IN as you alternate sides

Method

1. Lie on your back with your spine and hips in neutral. Engage your lower abdominals and slowly lift your legs to the ceiling. Place your hands behind your back to support you.

2. Lower one leg toward the mat, pointing your feet and lengthening your leg away from you. Raise your leg and repeat the movement with the opposite leg.

GOOD FOR:

Low-back pain

Patellofemoral pain

Patellar tendonitis

Achilles tendonitis

Adductor strain

Medial collateral ligament injury

Anterior cruciate ligament injury

Hamstring strain

Meniscus tear

Muscles

Lengthen

Quadriceps

Psoas

Levator scapulae

Rhomboids

Pectoralis major/minor

Hamstrings

Obliques

Tensor fasciae latae

Iliotibial band

Strengthen

Lower abdominals

Psoas

Obliques

Latissimus dorsi

Quadratus lumborum

Deep neck flexors

Posterior deltoid

Common mistakes to avoid

Don't lose control of your hips or let your abdominals relax.

Keep your feet lengthened.

Don't tense your neck; keep it relaxed.

Don't rely on your hips to support you and don't lose control of the height of the hips, by letting the abdominals relax.

Don't lose the lengthening position of your feet.

Shoulder challenge

SPORTS: BASEBALL, FOOTBALL, SAILING, SKIING, SWIMMING, WINDSURFING, TENNIS

Focus

To train the gluteals

To enhance stability in the trunk

To achieve coordination in the trunk, hips, thoracic spine and shoulder girdle

Muscles

Lengthen

Psoas

Quadriceps

Rectus abdominis

Strengthen

Gluteals

Abdominals

Hamstrings

Back extensors

Method

1. Sit on the floor with your knees bent, back resting against a fitness ball.

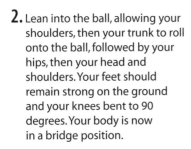

2. Lean into the ball, allowing your shoulders, then your trunk to roll onto the ball, followed by your hips, then your head and shoulders. Your feet should remain strong on the ground and your knees bent to 90 degrees. Your body is now in a bridge position.

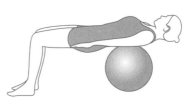

Variations

While you're in the bridge position, lift and straighten one leg. Raise your arms above your head and raise the opposite arm.

Common mistakes to avoid

Don't allow your hips to sink into the floor. Maintain your neutral pelvis position.

Don't arch your back or use your back to push down on the ball. The effort should come from your core.

> **GOOD FOR:**
>
> Swimmer's shoulder pain
> Swimmer's elbow
> Shoulder dislocation
> Tennis elbow
> Biceps tendonitis
> Acromioclavicular joint pain

Side kick series

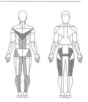

Focus

To create rotational control of the trunk

To stabilize hips

Breathe IN as you kick forward.
Breathe OUT as you lower your leg.

Method

1. Lie on one side and prop up your head onto your hand. Your whole body should be in a straight line. Place your other hand in front to help stabilize your body.

2. Engage your lower stomach muscles and inhale. Kick your top leg forward, making sure to keep your body stable and allowing your hips to conduct the movement. Exhale, drawing in your abdominals, and return to the starting position. Repeat.

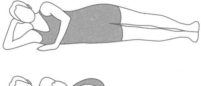
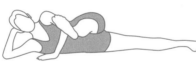

Muscles

Lengthen

Hip adductors

Gluteals

Calf muscles

Erector spinae

Strengthen

Hip abductors

Lower abdominals

Obliques

Quadratus lumborum

Scapular stabilizers

Tensor fasciae latae

Quadriceps

Variation

Raise the top leg parallel to the hip. Bring your foot in front of the bottom leg to touch the floor. Return to the center and lengthen the top leg behind you, touching the floor behind the bottom leg.

Common mistakes to avoid

Don't lose your core stability. Keep your trunk stable.

Don't push your chin forward. Ensure that your neck is aligned with your body.

Don't slump your hips or shoulders forward.

Don't move from the waist—the movement should be from your hips.

GOOD FOR:	
Ankle inversion injury	Swimmer's knee
Hamstring strain	Groin strain
Gluteal hip pain	Low-back pain
Shin splints	Patellofemoral pain
Stress fracture	Patellar tendonitis
Achilles tendonitis	Spondylolisthesis
Meniscus tear	Adductor strain
Swimmer's ankle	

Side rolls

SPORTS: FOOTBALL, GOLF, RUNNING, SAILING, SKIING, SOCCER, WINDSURFING

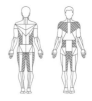

Focus

To rotate through the spine in a controlled motion

Breath IN to prepare. Breathe OUT on the outward movement and when returning your knees to neutral.

Muscles
Lengthen
Muscles in reverse

Strengthen
Obliques
Quadratus lumborum
Serratus anterior
Adductors
Tensor fasciae latae
Latissimus dorsi
Pectoralis major

Method

1. Lie on your back with your knees bent, feet together, pelvis in neutral, shoulder blades evenly on the floor. Place your hands at your sides, palms upward.

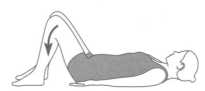

2. Engage the lower stomach muscles. Keeping your knees together, allow the knees to rotate to one side. Keep your shoulder blades on the floor. Bring your knees back to the neutral starting position. The rolling movement is a sequence through the waist, flowing through to the ribs and back.

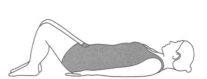

Variation

Repeat step one. Stretch the left leg out straight, and rotate your right knee to one side. Bring your knees back to the starting position and repeat on the opposite side.

Common mistakes to avoid

Don't allow the weight of your legs to pull you down as you lower your knees.

Don't lose your neutral pelvis position.

GOOD FOR:

Low-back pain
Adductor strain
Hamstring strain

Single leg stretch

SPORTS: BASEBALL, CYCLING, FOOTBALL, GOLF, HOCKEY, HORSE RIDING, RUNNING, SAILING, SKIING, SOCCER, SWIMMING, TENNIS, WINDSURFING

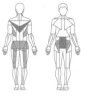

Focus

To achieve stability of movement

To coordinate the movement

To gain control of the deep abdominal muscles

Breathe IN to prepare. Breathe OUT on the outward movement.

Method

1 Lie on your back with your knees folded onto your chest. Your knees should be at 90 degrees, with your toes together and slightly pointed. Place your hands on the outside of your calves. Your head should be resting on the floor.

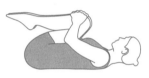

2. Engage your lower abdominals and slowly curl your head up. Place your right hand on the outside of your right ankle. Place your left hand on the inside of the right knee. Stretch your left leg away from your body keeping it parallel. Keep the foot soft. As you stretch your left leg away, fold your right knee closer to your chest.

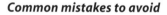

Common mistakes to avoid

Don't forget to keep your lower abdominals engaged throughout the movement.

Don't lose your neutral pelvis position.

Don't tense your neck and shoulders.

Don't lean toward one side. Keep the length even on both sides of your trunk.

Muscles

Lengthen

Hamstrings

Gluteals

Latissimus dorsi

Obliques

Quadratus lumborum

Strengthen

Abdominals

Deep neck flexors

Scapular stabilizers

Obliques

Quadratus lumborum

GOOD FOR:	
Shoulder pain	Low-back pain
Adductor strain	Anterior cruciate ligament injury
Ankle inversion injury	
Gluteal hip pain	Spondylolisthesis
Shin splints	Swimmer's knee
Stress fracture	Meniscus tear
Achilles tendonitis	Calf strain
Neck strain	Groin injuries
Patellofemoral pain	Hamstring strain

Sitting knee folds

SPORTS: BASEBALL, CYCLING, FOOTBALL, HOCKEY, HORSE RIDING, RUNNING
SAILING, SKIING, SOCCER, TENNIS, WINDSURFING

Focus

To improve the performance of the muscles that lift the leg towards the chest

To improve the control of the trunk muscles

To stretch the muscles in the back of the hip

Breathe IN to prepare. Breathe OUT to raise and lower your leg.

Muscle
Lengthen

Gluteals

Piriformi

Strengthen

Psoas

Transversus abdominis

Scapular stabilizers

Method

1. Sit on a chair with a straight back. Your hips should be at right angles to your trunk and shoulders in line with your hips. Knees should be bent and your feet placed evenly on the floor.

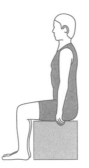 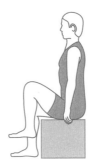

2. Place your hands lightly at your sides and allow one knee to raise from the chair. Don't use your hips to provide the movement, just allow your leg to float up. Return the leg to the starting position.

Variation

Repeat the same movement whilst standing. When the thigh is lifted, use your hands to place pressure on your thigh.

Common mistakes to avoid

Don't allow your back to move as you raise your leg.

Don't use your hips to pull the leg upward.

GOOD FOR:
Low-back pain
Achilles tendonitis
Hamstring strain
Gluteal hip pain
Medial collateral ligament injury
Anterior cruciate ligament strain
Meniscus tear
Piriformis pain

Superman

SPORTS: BASEBALL, CYCLING, GOLF, HOCKEY, HORSE RIDING, SAILING, SKIING, SWIMMING, TENNIS, WINDSURFING

Focus

To extend the spine

To create stability in the spine when extended

To strengthen the upper limbs

Breathe IN to prepare. Breathe OUT as you roll the ball forward.

Method

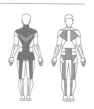

Muscles
Lengthen
Pectoralis major/minor
Rectus abdominis
Psoas
Quadriceps
Tibialis anterior
Scapular stabilizers

Strengthen
Middle/upper trapezius
Deep neck flexors
Hamstrings
Gluteals
Erector spinae
Lower trapezius

1. Kneel on a fitness mat with a fitness ball in front of you. Lean over the fitness ball, placing your hands on the floor. Your hands should be in line with your shoulders.

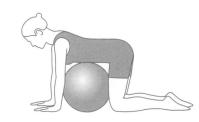

2. Push downward against the ball, rolling it forward until your arms are extended and your hips are touching the ball. Continue rolling the ball, extending the arms through the spine.

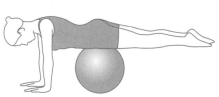

GOOD FOR:	
Shoulder dislocation	Hamstring strain
Biceps tendonitis	Swimmer's shoulder
Low-back pain	Spondylolisthesis
Shoulder pain	Swimmer's elbow
Acromioclavicular joint pain	Swimmer's knee
Neck strain	Muscle imbalance
	Golfer's elbow

Common mistakes to avoid

Don't lose control of the ball. Make sure the ball moves in a straight line.

Don't bend your arms.

Make sure your arms are extended fully as the ball is rolled.

Don't place any pressure onto your chest.

Swimming

SPORTS: BASEBALL, FOOTBALL, GOLF, HOCKEY, HORSE RIDING, RUNNING,
SAILING, SKIING, WINDSURFING

Focus

To stabilize the back extensors

To strengthen gluteals and hamstrings

To gain control through the deep stabilizing abdominal muscles

**Breathe IN to prepare. Breathe OUT as you lift your arm and leg.
Breathe IN as you lower them.**

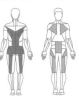

Muscles
Lengthen

Hip flexors

Pectoralis major/minor

Latissimus dorsi

Shoulder medial
rotators

Rectus femoris

Strengthen

Scapular stabilizers

Multifidis

Gluteals

Hamstrings

Back extensors

Deep neck flexors

Hip extensors

Method

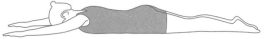

1. Lie face down on the floor, with your arms and legs extended,
shoulder-width apart. Your feet should be pointed and turned
outward. Place a small cushion under your forehead.

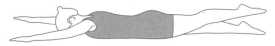

2. Lift your left leg and right arm up and away from you. Stretch your
fingers and toes out, feeling the space between each one. Release
the lift and allow your arms and legs to return slowly to the floor.

GOOD FOR:	
Low-back pain	Acromioclavicular joint pain
Piriformis pain	
Gluteal hip pain	Shoulder pain
Achilles problems	Biceps tendonitis
Adductor tendonitis	Patellofemoral pain
Shoulder dislocation	Medial collateral ligament injury
Rotator cuff pain	
Neck strain	Anterior cruciate ligament injury

Variations

Rest your head on your hands and raise only
your legs alternately.

When your arm and leg are raised, beat
them on the ground to the count of five.

Common mistakes to avoid

Don't lift or twist your lower back.

Don't lock your elbows out.

Don't lose tension in your foot.

Don't poke your chin out or tense your neck.

Teaser

SPORTS: BASEBALL, CYCLING, FOOTBALL, SAILING, SKIING, SWIMMING, TENNIS, WINDSURFING

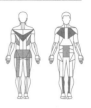

Focus

To maintain control of the deep abdominals

To achieve balance

Method

1. Sit in balance point position. Wrap your hands around your knees and lift your feet off the ground.

2. Extend both legs and stretch out your arms in front of you, so that they are parallel to your legs. Imagine a strong magnet is pulling the toes and fingers upward and away from you. If you lose your balance return to the starting position and repeat the exercise.

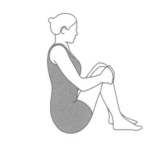

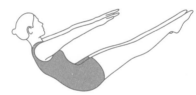

Muscles

Lengthen

Hamstrings

Rectus abdominis

Gluteals

Latissimus dorsi

Hip lateral rotators

Levator scapulae

Adductors

Strengthen

Abdominals

Scapular stabilizers

Tibialis anterior

Pectoralis major/minor

Abductors

Latissimus dorsi

Variations

To advance this movement, lift your arms up toward the ceiling, so that they are alongside your ears. Keep your shoulder blades pulled down your back. Pull your navel deep into your spine and begin slowly to roll your body back and forth on the mat.

Common mistakes to avoid

Don't lose your focus of your abdominals.

Don't lose the tension and alignment in your upper body.

Don't tense your neck.

Don't rush the movement. Move your legs slowly.

GOOD FOR:	
Hamstring strain	Swimmer's knee pain
Low-back pain	Muscle imbalance
Spondylolisthesis	Swimmer's ankle
Ankle inversion injury	Neck strain

Tennis ball raises

SPORTS: BASEBALL, CYCLING, FOOTBALL, HOCKEY, RUNNING, SKIING,
SOCCER, SWIMMING, TENNIS

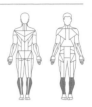

Focus

To achieve alignment between feet, ankles, knees, and hips

To strengthen the muscles around the ankles

To stabilize muscles around the ankles and bones

To improve static standing balance

Muscles
Strengthen

Tibialis posterior

Soleus

Gastrocnemius

Peroneus longus/brevis

Method

1. Stand in neutral position. Place a tennis ball between your ankles, just below the insides of your ankle bones. Use a wall as support if you need to.

2. Maintaining the length in your spine, breathe out and, tensing your abdominal muscles, bend your knees directly over your feet, keeping your heels firmly planted on the ground. Return to the starting position.

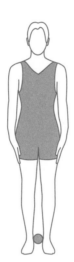
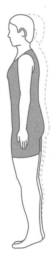

Common mistakes to avoid

Don't allow your bottom to stick out as you bend your knees.

Don't raise your heels from the ground.

Don't shift your weight to the sides of your feet.

GOOD FOR:	
Hip pain	Medial collateral ligament injury
Gluteal hip pain	
Meniscus tear	Anterior cruciate ligament injury
Hamstrings strain	
Calf muscle strain	Achilles tendonitis
Ankle inversion injury	Heel pain
Patellofemoral pain	Shin splints
	Stress fracture

Torpedo

SPORTS: BASEBALL, CYCLING, FOOTBALL, HOCKEY, HORSE RIDING, RUNNING, SAILING, SKIING, SOCCER, SWIMMING, TENNIS

Focus

To maintain control through the trunk, obliques and outer thighs

Breathe OUT as your raise your leg. Breathe IN to lower your leg.

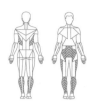

Muscles
Lengthen

Muscles on the
opposite side

Strengthen

Quadratus lumborum

Obliques

Tensor fasciae latae

Sternocleidomastoid

Latissimus dorsi

Abdominals

Tibialis anterior

Peroneus longus

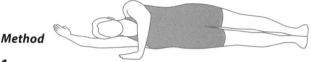

Method

1. Lie on your side, with your head resting on the lower arm. Place the top arm in front of your body with your palm facing downward, level with your chest. Keep your head in alignment with your body. Keep your shoulder blades pulled down your back and your waist open.

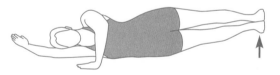

2. Contract your lower abdominals and allow the top leg then the bottom leg to rise, keeping them parallel to each other. Hold this position. Gently lower the bottom leg, then the top leg to return to starting position.

Common mistakes to avoid

Don't use your supporting arm to move your legs.

Don't tilt your pelvis.

Don't allow your waist to flop forward.

GOOD FOR:		
Low-back pain	Ankle inversion injury	Shoulder dislocation
Hip pain	Medial collateral ligament injury	Achilles tendonitis
Biceps tendonitis		Heel pain
Swimmer's shoulder	Anterior cruciate ligament injury	Gluteal hip pain
Spondylolisthesis		Adductor strain
Swimmer's ankle pain	Hamstring strain	Piriformis pain
Swimmer's knee	Acromioclavicular joint pain	

Waist twists in standing

SPORTS: BASEBALL, CYCLING, GOLF, RUNNING, SAILING, TENNIS, WINDSURFING

Focus

To rotate the trunk without moving the hips

Breathe OUT as you rotate out. Breathe IN as you return to the starting position.

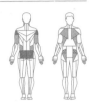

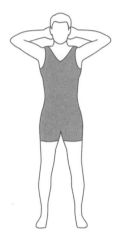
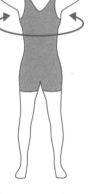

Muscles
Lengthen

Serratus anterior

Pectoralis

Quadratus lumborum

Triceps

Obliques

Strengthen

Obliques

Gluteals

Thoracic rotators

Deltoid

Method

1. Stand with your feet hip-width apart, pelvis in neutral. Your spine should be long. Place your hands behind your head, keeping your elbows wide, but not locked.

2. Engage your lower abdominal muscles and, keeping your chest open, rotate the upper trunk to the right. Take care to keep your arms steady, don't use them to lead the movement. Keep your hips facing forward throughout. Return to the starting position.

GOOD FOR:
Low-back pain

Common mistakes to avoid

Don't allow the hips to twist.

Don't push through the arms to achieve the movement.

Don't slump or lose height as you rotate. You need to remain tall throughout the movement.

Wrist strengthening

SPORTS: GOLF, HOCKEY, SWIMMING, TENNIS

Focus

To strengthen the wrist and forearm muscles

Method

1. Use a cord to tie a weight to a pole. Stand in neutral with abdominals strong and your feet hip-width apart. Hold the pole at waist height in front of you. Your wrist should be parallel to your forearm.

2. Rotate your right wrist in order to turn the pole so that the rope begins to wind itself around the pole. Once the rope has wrapped itself completely around the pole, reverse the wrist movement to unwind the rope. Lower the weight back to the floor. Repeat with the other wrist.

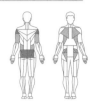

Muscles
Lengthen
Wrist flexors
Wrist extensors

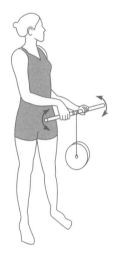

GOOD FOR:
Swimmer's elbow
Golfer's elbow
Tennis elbow

Common mistakes to avoid

Take care to rotate your wrist completely.

Keep your forearms parallel to the floor at all times.

Top-to-toe guide to injuries

Neck

Neck strain
Cycling
Skiing and snowboarding

Shoulder

Acromioclavicular joint sprain
Baseball
Hockey
Soccer

Joint subluxation
Baseball

Labrum damage
Baseball

Little pitcher's shoulder
Baseball

Rotator cuff pain
Baseball
Tennis

Shoulder dislocation
Football
Sailing and windsurfing
Skiing and snowboarding

Shoulder impingement
Basketball

Shoulder pain
Horse riding

Golfer's shoulder
Golf

Sailor's shoulder
Sailing and windsurfing

Swimmer's shoulder
Swimming

Arms and hands

Biceps tendonitis
Baseball
Sailing and windsurfing
Tennis

Golfer's elbow
Golf

Little leaguer's elbow
Baseball

Swimmer's elbow
Swimming

Tennis elbow
Tennis

Ulnar ligament tear
Hockey

Wrist injury
Skiing and snowboarding

Back

Back strain
Tennis

Low-back pain
Golf
Hockey
Horse riding
Sailing and windsurfing

Piriformis syndrome
Running

Swimmer's back
Swimming

Hips
Horse riding
Groin injuries
Soccer

Legs

Upper leg
Hamstring strain
Cycling
Football
Running

Iliotibial band strain
Cycling
Running

Tennis leg
Tennis

Knee

Anterior cruciate ligament injury
Basketball
Hockey
Skiing and snowboarding

Cycling knee pain
Cycling

Knee injury
Basketball
Hockey
Soccer

Medial collateral ligament injury
Football
Hockey
Skiing and snowboarding
Soccer

Meniscus tear
Football
Hockey
Soccer

Patellofemoral pain
Running
Sailing and windsurfing

Glossary of terms

Swimmer's knee
Swimming

Lower leg
Calf muscle strain
Basketball
Football
Running

Stress fracture
Running

Shin splints
Running
Soccer

Ankle
Ankle inversion injury
Basketball
Football
Hockey
Running
Sailing and windsurfing
Skiing and snowboarding
Soccer
Tennis

Achilles tendonitis
Baseball
Basketball
Cycling
Running
Tennis

Soccer ankle
Soccer

Swimmer's ankle
Swimming
Baseball

Foot
Plantar fasciitis
Running
Tennis

Abduction
A movement that draws away from the body.

Adduct
To move toward the body.

Adhesion
Abnormal adherence of collagen fibers to surrounding structures during immobilization following trauma or as a complication to surgery. Restricts normal elasticity of structures involved.

Anterior
The front or forward portion.

Anterior cruciate ligament (ACL)
A primary stabilizing ligament within the center of the knee joint that prevents hyperextension and excessive rotation of the joint.

Anti-inflammatory
Anything that reduces swelling or inflammation including ice and medication (aspirin, ibuprofen, etc.)

Bruise
A discoloration of the skin as a result of an extravasation of blood into the underlying tissues.

Bursa
A closed sac filled with fluid which eases the movement of muscles over

bones and muscle over muscles.

Cartilage
Tissue located between the ends of bones for cushioning and protection.

Centering and core stability
Engages the deep stabilizing muscles (transversus abdominis, pelvic floor and multifudis muscles) in order to stabilize (support) the lumbar spine.

Cervical spine
Part of the spine associated with the neck.

Clavicle
The collar bone, which connects the sternum (breastbone) to the scapula (shoulder blade).

Contusion
An injury to a muscle and tissues caused by a blow from a blunt object.

Disk
Material between the vertebrae which cushion against shock. The disk consists of a thick fiber ring which surrounds a soft gel-like interior.

Dislocation
Complete displacement of joint surfaces.

Extension
Straightening and moving the bones apart.

Fascia
A connective sheath consisting of fibers and fat which unites the skin to the underlying tissues.

Femur
Thigh bone.

Flexibility
Ability of the muscle to relax and yield to stretch and stress forces. Flexibility exercises consist of elongation of the soft tissue to prepare for the rigors of sport.

Flexion
A movement that bends, bringing bones together.

Girdle of strength
Term used by Joseph Pilates referring to the natural corset around the trunk.

Grade one injury
A mild injury in which ligament, tendon or other musculo-skeletal tissue may have been stretched or contused, but not torn.

Grade two injury
A moderate injury when tissue has been partially, but not totally, torn with appreciable limitation in function of the injured tissue.

Grade three injury
A severe injury in which tissue has been significantly or in some cases, totally torn, which causes a virtual loss of function of the injured tissue.

Humerus
Bone of the upper arm that runs from the elbow to the shoulder.

Hyperextension
Extreme extension of a limb or body part.

Iliotibial band
A thick, wide fascial layer that runs from the iliac crest of the pelvis to the knee joint and is occasionally inflamed as a result of excessive running.

Impingement
Pinching together of the supraspinatus muscle and other soft tissue in the shoulder, which is common in throwing, serving, and other sporting activities.

Inflammation
Joint inflammation is the body's reaction to various disease processes. These include mechanical injury to a joint (including a fracture), the presence of an infection (usually caused by bacteria or viruses), an attack on the joints by the body itself (an auto-immune disease), or accumulated "wear and tear" on joints. Inflammation shows itself through various degrees of pain, sweating, heat, redness, and/or loss of function.

Lateral
The outside portion of a particular body part.

Lateral collateral ligament (LCL)
Ligament of the knee attaching the lateral femoral condyle to the fibula head. It lies on the outside of the knee joint.

Ligament
Blend of fibrous tissue that attaches bone to bone.

Lumbar vertebrae
Five vertebrae of the lower back that articulate with the sacrum to form the lumbosacral joint.

Medial
The inside or center portion of the body.

Medial collateral ligament (MCL)
Ligament of the knee attaching the medial structure of the knee joint, including the patella and patellar tendon on the inside of the knee joint.

Meniscus
Crescent-shaped cartilage, usually pertaining to the knee joint. There are the medial and lateral meniscus and they absorb weight within the knee and provide stability.

Mobilizing muscles
The muscles responsible for large movements. These muscles turn on and off and are usually quite long. They are quick to tire and to feel fatigue.

Muscles
Tissues which contract when lengthened, extended, contracted, or flexed.

Nerve
One of many fibers or

bundles of fibers which form the neural system conveying impulses and sensations between the brain, the spinal cord, and all the parts of the body.

Neutral pelvis
The correct postural alignment of our pelvis, which helps to ensure the natural curves of the spine and good muscle balance.

Neutral spine
The correct postural alignment of the spine, maintaining the natural curves of the spine and promoting good muscle balance and ligament length throughout the spine.

Orthopedics
A field in medicine which focuses on the muscles, bones, and soft tissues.

Palpate
To touch or feel.

Patella
The kneecap. The patella protects the distal end of the femur as well as increasing the mechanical advantage and force generation of the quadriceps muscle group.

Patellofemoral joint
Articulation of the kneecap and the femur. Inflammation can occur from acute injury to the patella, overuse from excessive running, chronic wear and tear of the knee, and poor foot mechanics. In its worst form,

patellofemoral irritation can lead to chondromalacia, which may require surgery.

Pelvic stability
The ability to maintain the pelvis in its neutral position while the limbs are moving.

Physiotherapy
A type of treatment for injuries or disease through physical and mechanical means, utilizing ice, heat, massage, ultrasound, and exercise.

Plantar
Pertaining to the sole of the foot.

Plantar fascia
The tight band of tissue beneath the arch of the foot, connecting the heel and ball of the foot.

Posterior
The back or rear side of a muscle or other soft tissue.

Powerhouse
The term used by Joseph Pilates to identify the core stabilizing muscles.

Proprioception
Where the body functions at a very precise and controlled level.

Quadriceps
A group of four muscles of the front thigh that run from the pelvis and form a common tendon at the patella. Responsible for knee extension.

Scapula
The shoulder blade.

Sciatica
Irritation of the sciatic nerve resulting in pain or tingling running down the inside of the leg.

Sciatic nerve
A major nerve that carries impulses for muscular action and sensations between the low back and thigh and lower leg. It is the longest nerve in the body.

Slipped disk
Rupture of spinal disk causing the core of the disk to "slip" in to the spinal cord. This creates pain, numbing, and tingling in the muscles served by those affected nerves.

Stabilizer muscles
These muscles hold the bones in place so that movement can take place freely around the joint.

Sternum
The breast bone.

Spondylolisthesis
Usually caused by degenerative spinal disk disease and often affects women over 40 years of age.

Stretching
Any therapeutic maneuver designed to elongate shortened soft-tissue structures and thereby increase flexibility.

Supination
When the ankle appears to be "tipped" to the outside so

that you are standing on the outside border of the foot.

Talus
The ankle bone that articulates with the tibia and fibula to form the ankle joint.

Tendon
Tissue that connects muscle to bone.

Tendonitis
Inflammation, tearing, tightness, or weakness in the tendons attaching muscles to bones. Tendonitis can restrict or inhibit adduction, abduction, supination, etc.

Thoracic
Group of twelve vertebrae located in the thorax which articulate with the twelve ribs.

Thoracic or lateral breathing
Expansion of the lower rib cage during inhalation and contraction during exhalation. Increases oxygen intake and encourages correct use of the abdominals.

Tibia
Larger of the two bones of the lower leg and the weight-bearing bone of the shin.

Ultrasound
Electrical modality transmitting a sound wave through an applicator into the skin and to the soft tissue. The aim is to heat the local area to relax the injured tissue and disperse oedema.

Further Information

United States
Pilates Method Alliance
http://pilates.about.com

Santa Barbara Pilates Studio
http://sbpilates.com

United States Pilates Association
www.unitedstatespilatesassociation.com

USA Track and Field
www.usatf.org

United Kingdom
Pilates Foundation
www.pilatesfoundation.com

UK Sport
www.uksport.gov.uk

English Institute of Sport
www.eis2win.co.uk

Australia
Australian Pilates Method Association
www.australianpilates.asn.au

Sports
Baseball
www.mlb.com

Basketball
www.nba.com

Cycling
www.usacycling.org

Golf
www.usga.org

Hockey
www.usahockey.com

Horse riding
www.usef.org

Sailing and windsurfing
www.usasailing.org

Skiing and snowboarding
www.ussa.com

Soccer
www.ussoccer.com

Swimming
www.usaswimming.org

Tennis
www.usta.com

Index

Note: Bold page numbers refer to illustrations; *italics* refer to the Glossary